AF526877

Exam-Oriented SURGERY

QUESTIONS and ANSWERS

Exam-Oriented SURGERY

QUESTIONS and ANSWERS

K. Mukhopadhyay
MD, FCGP, PGCCHFWM
Associate Professor
College of Medicine and JNM Hospital
Kalyani, West Bengal

CBS

CBS Publishers & Distributors Pvt Ltd

New Delhi • Bengaluru • Pune • Kochi • Chennai

ISBN : 978-81-239-1930-0

First Edition : 2011
Reprint : 2013

Copyright © Publisher

All rights reserved. No part of this book may be reproduced or transmitted in any form or by any means, electronic or mechanical, including photocopying, recording, or any information storage and retrieval system without permission, in writing, from the publisher.

Published by Satish Kumar Jain and produced by V.K. Jain for
CBS Publishers & Distributors Pvt. Ltd.,
CBS Plaza, 4819/XI Prahlad Street, 24 Ansari Road, Daryaganj,
New Delhi - 110002, India. • Website: www.cbspd.com
e-mail: delhi@cbspd.com, cbspubs@airtelmail.in
Ph.: 23289259, 23266861, 23266867 • Fax: 011-23243014

Branches:

- ***Bengaluru:*** Seema House, 2975, 17th Cross, K.R. Road,
  Bansankari 2nd Stage, Bengaluru - 560070
  • Ph.: +91-80-26771678/79 • Fax: +91-80-26771680
  • E-mail: cbsbng@gmail.com, bangalore@cbspd.com
- ***Pune:*** Bhuruk Prestige, Sr. No. 52/12/2+1+3/2,
  Narhe, Haveli (Near Katraj-Dehu Road By-pass), Pune - 411041
  • Ph.: +91-20-64704058/59, 32342277 • E-mail: pune@cbspd.com
- ***Kochi:*** 36/14, Kalluvilakam, Lissie Hospital Road,
  Kochi - 682018, Kerala • Ph.: +91-484-4059061-65
  • Fax: +91-484-4059065 • E-mail: cochin@cbspd.com
- ***Chennai:*** 20, West Park Road, Shenoy Nagar, Chennai - 600030
  Ph.: +91-44-26260666, 26208620 • Fax: +91-44-42032115
  • E-mail: chennai@cbspd.com

Printed at :
India Binding House, Noida (UP)

Preface

SURGERY has developed tremendously during the last couple of decades like any other important branch of medical science. Its knowledge is required not only by the undergraduate/postgraduate students and surgeons, but also the general practitioner. I bestow my book Exam-Oriented Surgery to undergraduate students and general practitioners which is written in QUESTION and ANSWER format for quick review of the subject during exam period.

I remember my teachers Prof D Dey, Prof S Dey, Prof DK Roy, Prof SK Mallick, Dr D Dutta, Prof S Banerjee, Prof PK Choudhary, Dr S Roy, Dr S Mukherjee and Prof KK Choudhary whose lectures were of tremendous help in preparing the material for this book. I am thankful to Dr Bhaskar, Prof MK Das and Dr S. Mondu and grateful to those who encouraged me in writing this book. The help of Mr Ramanand Kumar Singh and Mr Umesh who typed the book is thankfully acknowledged.

The initiative of Mr Satish K Jain, Managing Director, and Mr YN Arjuna, Publishing Director, of CBS Publishers & Distributors is thankfully acknowledged in the publication of this book.

K. Mukhopadhyay

to

my teachers

Contents

Preface v

1. Shock and Blood Transfusion 1
2. Cyst 6
3. Acquired Immunodeficiency Syndrome 10
4. Ulcers, Sinus and Fistula 12
5. Transplantation 14
6. Laparoscopic Surgery 16
7. Wounds Infections, Gangrene and Tetanus 18
8. Nutrition 24
9. Burn 27
10. Warfare Injuries 31
11. Anaesthesia 33
12. Principles of Oncology 37
13. Day Surgery, Surgical Audit and Statistics 41
14. Basic Surgical Skills 44
15. Thyroid Gland 46
16. Parathyroid Gland 51
17. Adrenal Gland 53
18. Liver 57
19. Spleen 61
20. Gallbladder and Bile Duct 65
21. Pancreas 70
22. Oesophagus 77
23. Stomach and Duodenum 82
24. Peritoneum 90

25. Intestine (Small and Large) 97
26. Intestinal Obstruction 105
27. Vermiform Appendix 110
28. Rectum and Anal Canal 114
29. Hernia and Umbilicus 121
30. Urinary Symptoms : Anuria, Kidney 127
31. Urinary Bladder 136
32. Prostate and Seminal Vesicles 142
33. Urethra and Penis 148
34. Testis and Scrotum 151
35. Jaw, Lips, Palate, Face and Mouth 156
36. Salivary Gland 159
37. Neck 161
38. Chest 165
39. Cardiac Surgery 168
40. Breast 173
41. Diseases of Bones and Joints 179
42. The Foot 184
43. Osteomyelitis 186
44. Bone Tumours 190
45. Fracture and Dislocations 196
46. Fractures of Superior and Inferior Extremity 201
47. Problems of Shoulder and Elbow 209
48. Spine and Spinal Cord Injury 213
49. Head Injury 216
50. Postoperative Care 223

1 Shock and Blood Transfusion

LAQ 1 Define shock. What are the types of shock? How it manifests?

The word shock derived from Dutch word *schokken* means jolt or jerk. It is defined as a state of profound haemodynamic and metabolic disturbances, characterised by low perfusion, circulatory insufficiency leading to an imbalance between metabolic needs of vital organs and supply.

Types of shock

1. Hypovolemic or oligaemic shock
   - External haemorrhage
   - Internal haemorrhage
   - Burns, vomiting, diarrhoea
2. Cardiogenic shock
   - Intrinsic (myocardial damage)
   - Extrinsic embarrassment of cardiac function (cardiac temponade)
3. Vascular shock (altered peripheral vasomotor tone)
   - Neurogenic
   - Septic (severe gram-negative and positive infections)
   - Anaphylaxis

In vascular shock

(a) Peripheral pooling of blood increases
(b) Vascular permeability increases
(c) There is disseminated intravascular coagulation

Phases of hypovolemic shock

(i) Phase of compensation
(ii) Phase of decompensation

Neuroendocrine response of shock

- Release of ATCH, GH, ADH, β endorphin, dynorphin, cortisol, glucagon

Different mediators of septic shock

- Activation of complement systems
- Cytokines
- Platelet activating factors
- Products of arachidonic acid metabolism (PG, TXA_2, leukotrienes)
- Lysosomal enzyme

Clinical features of shock

Hypovolemic shock

- Cold clammy skin
- Oliguria
- Confusion
- Tachycardia
- Sweating
- Hypotension
- Acidosis
- Tachypnoea
- JVP falls

Cardiogenic shock

- Raised JVP
- Basal crepts
- Gallop rhythm

Septic shock

- Fever and rigor
- Bounding pulse
- Jaundice
- Coma
- Sign of DIC

Anaphylactic shock

- Urticaria
- Bronchospasm
- Low BP
- Warm peripheries
- Oedema of face, pharynx; larynx

Monitoring shock patient

(i) Central venous pressure (CVP)
(ii) Pulmonary artery wedge pressure by Swan-Ganz catheter
(iii) Intraarterial pressure
(iv) Chest X-ray
(v) Cardiac out put
(vi) Urine out put
(vii) Serial blood gas analysis
(viii) ECG.

Treatment of shock

(i) Adequate oxygenation, may require tracheostomy, endotracheal tube
(ii) Treat primary cause (stop haemorrhage; drain pus, etc.)
(iii) Improve ventricular filling by fluid replacement (crystalloid or colloids)
(iv) Improve cardiac contractility by dopamine or dobutamine
(v) Correct acid-base balance
(vi) In case of septic shock after improving hypovolemia, give suitable antibiotic, treat diabetes simultaneously with insulin, if diabetic.

(vii) Anaphylactic shock with adrenaline, corticosteroids and antihistaminics.
(viii) Vasodilators: After correction of hypovolemia, give hydralazine, phentolamine, chlorpromazine, nitroglycerine, etc. to increase tissue perfusion with caution

LAQ 2 What do you mean by multiorgan failure?

The impaired tissue oxygenation and microcirculatory abnormalities in case of irreversible shock causes damage of vital organs to produce multiple organ failure.

Insults of multiple organ dysfunction syndromes (MODS) are:

Primary insults	Compounding insults
Infection Trauma or surgery Burns Pancreatitis	Anoxia Hypovolemia Hospital infection Endotoxin, Malnutrition Hyperglycaemia Hyperthermia

Systemic inflammatory response in MODS are due to:

(i) Increased production of cytokines
(ii) Activation of coagulation and complements
(iii) Neutrophil degranulation and production of free radicals
(iv) Abnormal synthesis of nitric oxide.

LAQ 3 Classify haemorrhage.

It may be classified as:

According to site of origin

- **Arterial:** Bright red; spurting
- **Venous:** Dark red; steady copious flow
- **Capillary:** Bright red oozing

According to time and etiology

- **Primary:** At the time of trauma
- **Reactionary:** Within 24 hours due to slipping of ligature
- **Secondary:** After 7–14 days, due to infection of wall of blood vessels

According to nature

- **Revealved or external**
- **Concealed or internal**

SAQ 4 What are different important blood groups?

The different important blood groups are:

- Group A serum contains anti-B antibodies
- Group B serum contains anti-A antibodies
- Group AB serum contains none antibodies to A or B
- Group O serum contains antibodies to A and B both
- Rhesus Group positive and negative
- M, N, H, etc. are the other important blood groups.

LAQ 5 Mention the adverse reaction associated with transfusion of blood and blood components.

Adverse reaction of blood transfusion

Acute transfusion reaction

(i) Allergic reaction
(ii) Febrile non-haemolytic transfusion reaction
(iii) Anaphylactic reaction
(iv) Acute haemolytic transfusion reaction
(v) Transfusion related acute lung injury
(vi) Massive transfusion may lead to:
- Bleeding complication
- Hypocalcaemia and hypokalaemia
- pH abnormalities
- Hypothermia
- Acute respiratory distress syndrome

Delayed transfusion reactions

(i) Delayed transfusion reaction
(ii) Post-transfusion graft-versus-host disease
(iii) Transfusion transmitted diseases:
- Hepatitis B, C
- HIV
- CMV
- Syphilis
- Malaria
- Creutzfeldt-Jokob disease

SAQ 6 What are the principles of transfusion therapy?

(i) Chose the transfusion material which best supplies patients need
(ii) Anticipate therapeutic benefit versus risk
(iii) Most important contraindication is absence of specific indications.

LAQ 7 How an acute haemolytic reaction presents?

It presents with:

- Fever
- Chest pain
- Renal failure
- Haemoglobinuria
- Chill a rigor
- Dyspnoea
- DIC
- Nausea
- Restlessness
- Bleeding along surgical incision site
- Vomiting
- Hypotension

LAQ 8 What are the indications of following transfusion: (i) Whole blood, (ii) Packed RBC, (iii) Washed RBC, (iv) Leucocyte-reduced RBC, (v) Irradiated RBC, (vi) Plasma-derived volume expanders, (vii) Platelet transfusion, (viii) Granulocyte transfusion?

(i) **Whole blood**: Patient requiring oxygen carring capacity and intravascular replacement, viz. haemorrhage, surgery, exchange transfusion.

(ii) **Packed blood**: Symptomatic anaemia.

(iii) **Washed blood**: PNH; IgA deficiency patients.

(iv) **Leukocyte reduced RBC**: Preventing non-haemolytic transfusion reaction; preventing CMV infection; patient receiving multiple transfusion.

(v) **Plasma-derived volume expanders**: (i) Large volume plasma paracentesis, (ii) initial 24 hours of thermal injury.

(vi) **Platelet transfusion**: To prevent active bleeding associated with qualitative and quantitative deficiency of platelets.

(vii) **Granulocyte transfusion**: Patient with neutropenia ($<100/\mu L$) with gram-negative septicaemia or progressive soft tissue infection despite antibiotic therapy.

2 Cyst

SAQ 1 Define cyst.

Cysts are swelling generally lined by epithelium or endothelium, containing fluid. Its Greek origin means bladder. Greek "*Kustis*" means bladder.

LAQ 2 What are the different types of cysts?

The cysts may be lined by epithelium or endothelium called true cysts or false cysts due to collection of exudation or degeneration.

It may be classified as following:

Congenital

- **Sequestration** (dermoid)
- **Tubo-embryonic** (e.g. thyroglossal or postanal dermoid)
- **Cysts of embryonic remnants** e.g.: Cyst of urachus

Acquired

- **Retention cyst** (e.g. Bartholin's or sebaceous glands)
- **Distension cyst** (e.g. cystic hygroma)
- **Exudation cyst** (e.g. hydrocele, bursa)
- **Cystic tumours** (e.g. dermoid cysts of ovary)
- **Implantation dermoid**
- **Traumatic** (e.g. haematoma turning to cyst)
- **Degeneration**

Parasitic

Hydatid cyst

SAQ 3 How a cyst clinically presents?

Cyst's presentation

(i) It is smooth spherical
(ii) Fluctuating
(iii) Transilluminating
(iv) A cyst may be hard if tense with fluid or may be confused with lipoma or cold abscess (also shows fluctuation). A calcified cyst may be transillumination negative.

SAQ 4 What are the effects and complications of a cyst?

The effects of cyst depend upon site and size. Complications may be:

- Infection
- Haemorrhage
- Torsion
- Calcification
- Cachexia

SAQ 5 What is dermoid cyst? How is it treated?

These epidermoid cysts are lined by epithelium and contain epithelial secretions.

Types

Congenital

- Sequestration dermoid
- Tubulodermoid
- Teratodermoids of ovary or testis

Cysts are treated by excision

Acquired

- Implantation dermoid

LAQ 6 Write short notes on sebaceous cyst.

These are retention cysts obstructing sebaceous duct; present in sites with sebaceous glands, viz. scalp; face, scrotum.

Complications:

- Infection
- Sebaceous horn
- Ulceration
- Calcification
- Cocks's peculiar tumour
- Malignancy (adenocarcinoma rarely)

Treatment

(i) Excision
(ii) Incision or avulsion
(iii) In scrotum, a single sebaceous cyst is excised if there are more than one cysts, scrotal skin with cyst are removed. For multiple scrotal sebaceous cysts, testes are placed in thigh pocket and whole scrotal skin is cut.

SAQ 7 What is hydatid cyst?

This a parasitic cyst produced by *Echinococcus granulosus* which completes its life cycle in dog (definitive host); sheep or man (occasionally) as intermediate host.

Sites are: Liver (1st filter); lungs (2nd filter), brain (3rd filter)

Structure of cyst:

1. Ectocyst
2. Endocyst covered with:
    (a) Laminated membrane
    (b) Germinal layer
    (c) Brood capsules

Cyst contains: (i) fluid, (ii) hydatid cyst, and (iii) daughter cysts

SAQ 8 What complications may arise out of hydatid cysts?

Complications of hydatid cyst:

(i) Rupture
(ii) Calcification
(iii) Suppuration
(iv) Anaphylaxis

SAQ 9 How to diagnose hydatid cyst?

Diagnosis of hydatid cyst

(i) Eosinophilia in blood
(ii) Casoni's test
(iii) Complement fixation and other serological tests
(iv) ELISA
(v) Cyst on X-ray or USG; CT; MRI

LAQ 10 How to treat Hydatid cyst?

Treatment of hydatid cyst

Medical

(i) Mebendazole 40–50 mg/kg/day or
(ii) Albendazole 400 mg BD or 10–15 mg/kg × 3 months
(iii) Praziquantal for pulmonary cyst 40 mg/kg/day in two divided doses

Postoperative albendazole and praziquantal for 2 weeks

Surgical

For uncomplicated liver cyst as PAIR, i.e. puntcure; aspiration; injection, reabsorption or cystotomy or partial cystectomy with drainage

For children

(i) Deroofing plus tube drainage
(ii) Capitonnage
(iii) Omentoplasty
(iv) Pericystectomy

LAQ 11 What are the indications; contraindications and complications of puncture aspiration injections and resorptions, i.e. PAIR surgery?

PAIR Surgery

Indications	Contraindications	Complications
(i) Refusal of surgery (ii) Inoperable case (iii) Cyst more than 5 cm diameter and multiple cyst of 5 cm diameter (iv) Relapse cyst (v) No response to medications	(i) Multiple septed cyst (ii) Lung or bone cyst (iii) Dead or inactive cyst (iv) Hazardous location of cyst	(i) Urticaria (ii) Anaphylaxis (iii) Haematoma (iv) Fever (v) Biliary fistula (vi) Shock

SAQ 12 How to treat hydatid cyst in: (a) Lungs, (b) kidney, (c) spleen, (d) bone, (e) brain (f) muscle?

Lungs	Kidney	Spleen	Bone	Brain	Muscle
• Enucleation • Capitonnage • Lobectomy • Pneumonec-tomy	• Cystectomy • Marsupiali-sation • Nephrec tomy	• Splenectomy	• Wide resec-tion • Benzimida-zole chemo-therapy	• Cyst removed by Dowling technique	• Radical surgery or PAIR

3 Acquired Immunodeficiency Syndrome

LAQ 1 What is the causative organism of AIDS?

AIDS is caused by slow virus (lentivirus) of family retrovirus which is more closely related to non-human retrovirus producing simian immune deficiency syndrome of monkeys and distantly related to human T cell lymphocytotropic virus.

LAQ 2 Describe in brief HIV.

It is retrovirus with RNA with reverse transcriptase. The cell surface protein is GP_{120}. Function of GP_{120} is to recognize and bind to receptors particularly to CD4+ lymphocyte. Reverse transcriptase transcribes viral RNA to DNA.

Functional impairment of CD4+ lymphocyte produces:

(i) Impaired antibody formation
(ii) Disorder hypersensitivity
(iii) Disorder macrophage function.

LAQ 3 What is HAART therapy?

HAART stands for highly active antiretroviral therapy.

LAQ 4 How is AIDS transmitted?

Transmission of AIDS:

(i) Homosexual and hetrosexuals practicing oral sex
(ii) Drug addicts
(iii) Haemophiliacs receiving blood transfusion
(iv) Sub-Saharan Africans
(v) Patient to patient by surgical instruments or surgeon to patient or patient to surgeon. 1 ml of HIV-1 contaminated blood containing 50 HIV-I particles, while hepatitis B particles 10^9.

LAQ 5 How an HIV patient presents to a surgeon?

The surgeon's help required in the following situations in AIDS:

(i) Colorectal cancer or infection
(ii) Splenectomy for thrombocytopenia
(iii) Lymph node biopsy
(iv) Venous access to facilitate chemotherapy for infection

SAQ 6 What is Castleman's disease?

Genomic incorporation of Kaposi virus (herpes virus 8) encoding cytokine interleukin (IL6) resulting B cell, lymphoproliferation named after pathologist Benzamine Castleman of MIT, USA called Castleman's disease presents with hypersplenism, sequestration of platelets by spleen. Splenectomy helpful for thrombocytopenia.

4 Ulcers, Sinus and Fistula

SAQ 1 What is an ulcer?

It is discontinuity in continuity of epithelial surface with or without superadded infection.

SAQ 2 What are the things to be noted in ulcer?

Following things to be noted in ulcer:

- Site
- Size
- Shape
- Edge
- Base
- Discharge
- Lymph node draining if biopsy or serology
- Pain and tenderness
- General survey

SAQ 3 What is the principle of management of ulcer?

(i) Find out the etiology and assess ulcer properly
(ii) Correct co morbid factors and treat them.
(iii) Drain and desloughing
(iv) Dressing

SAQ 4 What is sinus and fistula?

Sinus is blind ending tract, lined by granulation tissue, leads from an epithelial surface. Congenital sinuses arise from congenital remnants of embryonic duct.

Fistula: It is a track connecting two epithelium-lined surfaces.

SAQ 5 What are the types of pathological sinuses?

It may be:

(a) Congenital (preauricular, umbilical, urachal, etc.)
(b) Acquired (pilonidal, actinomyces, tuberculosis, osteomyelitis, etc.)

SAQ 6 Write short notes on ranula.

Ranula: It is cystic swelling due to retention of glands (Blandin and Nuhn) of floor of the mouth like belly of a frog. Common in child in one side of frenum. It is mobile, bluish, transilluminant. It may be dissecting between mylohyoid muscle. Inside fluid is jelly-like. Treated by excision or partial excision with marsupialisation.

5 Transplantation

SAQ 1 Who first transplanted kidney; liver; and heart?

Joseph Murray transplanted kidney first amongst identical twins (1954) in Boston, USA. Tom Starzl in 1963 first transplanted liver.

Christiaan Barnard in 1967 first transplanted heart in Cape Town, South Africa.

SAQ 2 Define the following types of graft: (i) Allograft, (ii) Isograft, (iii) Orthotopic graft, (iv) Heterotopic graft, (v) Xenograft.

Allograft: Organ or tissue transplanted from one to another.

Isograft or syngeneic graft: Transplantation between twins of identical nature.

Orthotopic graft: Graft placed in normal site.

Heterotopic graft: Graft placed in different sites of normal position.

Xenograft: Graft between different species.

SAQ 3 What are different antigens responsible for allograft rejection?

(i) ABO blood group
(ii) Human leukocyte antigen (HLA), (major histocompatibility antigen)
(iii) Minor histocompatibility antigen, viz. polymorphic proteins which are less important

LAQ 4 What are the different types of allograft rejection?

These are:

Hyperacute graft rejection	Acute rejection	Chronic rejection
• Immediate • Characterised by intra-vascular thrombosis	• Occurs within 6 months • Characterised by intra-vascular mononuclear cell infiltration	• After 6 months of graft placement • Immunological • Myointimal cell proliferation in arteries, causing ischaemia and fibrosis

LAQ 5 Describe the mechanism of graft rejection.

T cells undergo clonal expansion after getting alloantigens, dependent on interleukin 2 and T cell growth factors. CD8 cells recognize donor HLA class I antigen to cause the death of target cells by lytic molecules like perforin and granzyme. HLA class II antigen causes direct tissue damage. CD4T cells produce B lymphocyte to differentiate into plasma cells to produce alloantibodies which binds to graft antigen to produce tissue injury by antibody-dependent, cell-mediated cytotoxicity or directly.

SAQ 6 Mention the important risk factors of chronic renal graft rejection.

- Earlier acute rejection
- Long cold ischaemic time
- Poor immunosuppression
- Poor HLA matching
- Raised blood lipids
- CMV infection

SAQ 7 Name the different immunosuppressive therapies.

(a) **Calcineurin blockers** (cyclosporin; tacrolimus)
(b) **Antiproliferative agents** (azathioprine, mycophenolate, mofatil)
(c) **Steroids** – glucocorticoids
(d) **Antibody therapies**: Antilymphocyte globulin; antilymphocyte serum
(e) **Rapamycin**: Arrest T cells division in G_1 phase

SAQ 8 Mention the important complications of immunosuppression.

(i) Infection (bacterial, viral, protozoal, fungal)
(ii) Malignancy.

SAQ 9 What are the signs of brainstem death?

(i) Absence of cranial nerve reflexes (viz. corneal, papillary, pharyngeal gag; tracheal cough; occulo vestibular caloric)
(ii) Absence of motor response.
(iii) Absence of spontaneous respirations.

SAQ 10. What are the major problems of organ transplantion?

(i) Shortage of organs
(ii) Graft rejection
(iii) Side effects of immunosuppression.

May be controlled by noval immunosuppression; stem cells tissue engineering; donor specific immunological tolerance and xenotransplantation.

6 Laparoscopic Surgery

SAQ 1 What are the advantages of laparoscopic surgery?

(i) Minimal tissue damage
(ii) Cost-effective
(iii) Short operation times and hospital stay
(iv) Faster recuperation
(iv) Less pain

SAQ 2 What are the disadvantages of open surgery?

- High morbidity
- Wound infection
- Bleeding
- Dehiscence
- Herniation
- Prolong recovery time
- Chest infection
- Deep vein thrombosis

SAQ 3 What are the disadvantages of minimal access surgery?

The disadvantages of minimal access surgery are:

- Difficulty in bleeding control and extraction of large specimens.
- Done by instruments so no tactile feedback and dependent on hand-eye co-ordination
- Remote operations and dependence on new techniques.

LAQ 4 What preoperative evaluation should be done before laparoscopic surgery?

Pt. fit for operations | **Informed consent** | **Operative difficulties should be predicted**

- Overall fitness
- Cardiac arrhythmia
- Previous surgery
- Coagulation
- Thromboprophylaxis
- Obesity
- Skeletal deformity
- Emphysema

SAQ 5 What are the intraoperative surgical principles of symptomatic gallstone disease? What operative complications may arise out of it?

Laparoscopic cholecystectomy is gold standard treatment of symptomatic gallstone disease. Following precautious should be taken:

(i) Meticulous creation of pneumoperitoneum by open or closed methods
(ii) Proper dissection and exposure of operative field
(iii) Control bleeding and prevent damage of organs
(iv) Postoperative care (perforation of gallbladder and bleeding is common.)

7 Wounds Infections, Gangrene and Tetanus

LAQ 1 Mention the risk factors for wound infection.

In normal person, infection is prevented by low gastric pH, antibodies, macrophages, neutrophils, lymphocytes.

The risks of wound infections are:

(i) Malnutrition and obesity
(ii) Diabetes, uraemia, jaundice
(iii) AIDS; radio- and chemotherapy
(iv) Shock
(v) Foreign bodies or haematoma
(vi) Colonisation of bacteria
(vii) Poor surgical technique (dead space)

SAQ 2 What were the contributions of the following medical professionals in wound infection?

(i) I. Semmelweiss: Mentioned about puerperal sepsis (1818–1865)
(ii) (a) GA Fleming
(b) HW Florey discovered pencillin
(c) EB Chain
(iii) HCJ Gram: Described Gram stain
(iv) Robert Koch: Koch's postulate (1843–1912)
(v) Louis Pasteur: Used antiseptics

SAQ 3 What do you mean by: (i) SIRS, (ii) SSSI, (iii) MODS, (iv) MSOF?

SIRS : Systemic inflammatory response syndrome
SSSI : Superficial surgical site infection
MODS : Multiple organ dysfunction syndrome
MSOF : Multiple system organ failure

SAQ 4 What do you mean by major wound infection?

(i) Major wound infection produces significant pus requiring draining, with systemic signs of tachycardia, pyrexia, neutrophilia.
(ii) Delayed return to home.

LAQ 5 What do you mean by ASEPSIS WOUNDS score?

A	S	E	P	S	I	S
Additional treatment by antibiotic Debridement Drainage	Serious discharge	Erythema	Purulent exudate	Separation from deep tissues	Isolation of bacteria	Stay in hospital prolong

SAQ 6 What are the different types of wound infections encountered in surgery?

These are:
(i) Wound abscess
(ii) Cellulitis
(iii) Lymphangitis
(iv) Bacteraemia
(v) Septicaemia
(iv) Specific wound infections, viz. gas gangrene, tetanus, etc.

SAQ 7 Name some antiseptics used in surgical practices.

These are:
(i) Chlorhexidine
(ii) Povidone-iodine
(iii) Cetrimide
(iv) Ethyl and isopropyl alcohol
(v) Hypochlorites (eusol milton)
(vi) Hexachlorophane

SAQ 8 Name some bacteria involved in wound infections.

(i) *Staphylococci*
(ii) *Streptococci*
(iii) *Clostridia*
(iv) Aerobic gram-negative (*Klebsiella; Proteus; E.coli; Pseudomonas*)
(v) *Bacteroides*

SAQ 9 Name some antimicrobials used for wound infections.

(i) Penicillin
(ii) Floxacillin
(iii) Methicillin
(iv) Mezlocillin and Azlocillin
(v) Cephalosporins
(vi) Aminoglycosides
(vii) Vancomycin
(viii) Imidazoles (metronidazole)
(ix) Carbapenems (meropenem, imipenem, ertapenem)

LAQ 10 What is gas gangrene? What are the causative organisms responsible for it?

Gas gangrene is infective gangrene caused by anaerobic saccharolytic (*Cl. welchii, Cl. septicum; Cl. edematiens*) and proteolytic bacteria (*Cl. sporogenes*) characterized by collection of gas in the muscles and subcutaneous tissues predisposed by:

(i) Lacerated wound
(ii) Poor drainage of wounds
(iii) Impaired circulations
(iv) Diabetes
(v) Presence of blood clots. Calcium foreign bodies, etc. predisposes its formation
(vi) Aerobic bacteria, etc. predisposes its formation.

Types: (i) Single muscle type, (ii) group type, (iii) massive type, (iv) fulminating type

LAQ 11 How to treat gas gangrene?

After confirming diagnosing by swab tested by microscope and X-ray showing gas shadows. It is treated as following:

Medically

(i) Suitable antibiotics
(ii) AGS polyvalent (IM)
(iii) Treat diabetes if presents
(iv) Blood transfusion
(v) Hyperbaric oxygen

Surgically

(i) Remove all foreign bodies
(ii) Devitalized tissues and blood clots
(iii) Damaged muscles

LAQ 12 What is tetanus? How it presents?

Tetanus is local infection caused by *Cl. tetani* causing general toxaemia and effect on motor centres in spinal cord and medulla. The organism is gram-positive, slender rod with terminal spores having drumstick appearance.

Clinical presentation:

- Malaise
- Tachycardia
- Risus sardonicus
- Opisthotonus
- Asphyxia
- Fever
- Lock jaw
- Dysphagia
- Generalized convulsion
- Rupture of muscle may occur

LAQ 13 What are the types of tetanus?

Types of tetanus:

- Tetanus neonatorum (in newborn)
- Latent tetanus wound is unrecognized
- Local tetanus (involving segments)
- Cephalic tetanus (involving head; hand)
- Bulbar tetanus (involves muscles of respiration and deglutination)
- Late tetanus (prolong incubation period)

LAQ 14 How will you treat tetanus?

(i) Passive immunization (equine or horse serum or ATG)
(ii) Antibiotics—pencillin
(iii) Care of the wound—all patients should receive active immunization after treatment cure
(iv) Symtomatic:— (a) Anticonvulsant; (b) muscle relaxants; (c) Ryles tube feeding

SAQ 15 What are the causes of death in tetanus?

(i) Lung causes aspiration; lack of ventilation; embolism
(ii) Hyperthermia
(iii) Co-existing diseases, complications.

LAQ 16 Write short note on keloid.

The word Kele means tumour, but it is not malignant. It is excessive overgrowth of scar tissue. It may spread to normal tissues. It may grow even after 6 months, whereas hypertrophic scar never grows. It is common in Negroes, female and patient with tuberculosis.

Histologically, fibroma with hyaline connective tissues. It never turns malignant. Scars of burns, vaccination, tuberculous sinus may turn keloid. Some people are keloid prone.

It is raised from surface, shiny pinks, with finger-like growing edges, may be with ulcers at margin with itching.

Treatment

- Application of corticosteroid ointment
- Intrakeloid injections of hydrocortisone
- Radiotherapy or intrakeloid excision
- Vitamin A high doses

SAQ 17 What do you mean by primary healing, secondary healing, tidy wounds and untidy wounds?

Primary healing occurs with clean wound edges. The ***secondary healing*** produces scar to draw skin edges in infected wound.

Tidy wounds are by sharp cuts. ***Untidy wounds*** are by crush or tearing containing devitalized tissue. It has to be converted to tidy wounds before healing.

SAQ 18 What is the best dressing?

As per Lister, skin is the best dressing.

SAQ 19 Mention in brief the steps of healing of wound.

Wound → coagulation → inflammation → angiogenesis → proteoglycan synthesis → epithelialization → remodelling.

SAQ 20 What is wound excision?

The untidy wound has to be excised also called untidy excision or debridement, alone under anaesthesia (local/regional/general) with bloodless field for identification (with adrenaline or tourniquet). Skin to be excised is marked with pen and from superficial to deeper layer. The devitalized dermis is pink. The devitalized tissue is excised. The radical wound excision is called pseudotumour approach.

LAQ 21 What are the different types of wounds.

Wounds may be:

(i) Bruise, contusion, haematoma
(ii) Bites
(iii) Puncture
(iv) Abrasion
(v) Friction
(vi) Burns
(vii) Laceration
(viii) Traction
(ix) Avulsion
(x) Crush
(xi) Fracture
(xii) Penetrating
(xiii) Injury to internal organs
(xiv) Gunshot injuries

SAQ 22 What is compartment syndrome?

In compartment syndrome, there is pain which is worse by passive stretching of the affected muscle, the product of degradation of muscle pour into bloodstream, blocks glomeruli producing myoglobinuria. Fasciotomy longitudinal along with longitudinal release of skin is advisible.

LAQ 23 What do you mean by ideal and adverse scar?

The differences between ideal and adverse scars are following:

Ideal scar	Adverse scar
(i) Clean incised edges without tissue loss (ii) Primary healing (iii) Minimal tension	(i) Wrongly directed (ii) Poorly alignment (iii) Stretched (iv) Contracted (v) Altered pigment, contour changes (vi) Tatoo or hypertrophic or stitch marks or keloid

8 Nutrition

SAQ 1 What physiological changes occur after starvation?

The physiological changes after 12 hours fastings are:

(i) Insulin level falls; glucagon level rises
(ii) Liver produces glucose
(iii) Muscle glycogen breaks to lactate (glycogenolysis)
(iv) Gluconeogenesis from sketetal muscle protein
(v) Prolong fasting produces ketone bodies form FA
(vi) Fat stores produce glycerol
(vii) Engery requirement declines due to decreased conversion of T_4 to T_3 hormones.

SAQ 2 What adoptive changes occur to injury and infection?

(i) Increased energy and nitrogen requirement
(ii) Plasma insulin level falls initially with counter regulatory hormone response of adrenaline, noradrenaline, glucagons and growth hormones
(iii) Insulin resistance causing glucose intolerance
(iv) Fluid retention
(v) Hypoalbuminaemia
(vi) Ketogenesis

SAQ 3 What are the nutritional requirement in healthy human?

Principal nutritional requirements are:

(i) Energy yielding foods: Carbohydrate, protein, fats
(ii) Trace elements
(iii) Vitamins
(iv) Minerals

SAQ 4 How to assess nutritional requirement?

(i) Body weight and anthropometric technique
(ii) Clinical weight and functional technique
(iii) Laboratory assessments

SAQ 5 Where to give nutritional support?

Nutritional support should be considered in:
(i) Malnurished patient with metabolic stress
(ii) Unable to take adequate nutrition for 5 days.

SAQ 6 What happens if patient with severe infection given 20% glucose as TPN?

Patients with severe infection if given 20% glucose there will be hyperglycaemia, they should be given liquid-based feeding regimen, which will provide energy. Higher glucose containing TPN should be avoided in patient in respirator.

LAQ 7 What are indications; contraindications of enteral and perenteral feeding?

Enteral feeding

Indications
- PEM
- Dysphagia
- Trauma
- To enhance adaptations after enterectomy

Contraindications
- Diarrhoea
- Ileus
- Proximal intestinal fistula
- Pancreatitis

Parenteral feeding

Indications
- Intestinal resection
- Ileus
- Pancreatitis
- Fistula

LAQ 8 What are the complications of enteral and perenteral nutrition?

Complications

Enteral
- Malposition and dislodgement of feeding tube
- Aspiration; fistula tube
- Peritonitis

(Complications of tube)

- Obstruction
- Diarrhoea, vomiting
- Hyperglycaemia
- Intestinal infection

Parenteral
- Embolism, • Catheter infection
- Pneumothorax • Endocarditis
- Thrombosis of veins
- Hyper- or hypoglycaemia • Acidosis
- Electrolyte imbalance
- Deficiency of vitamins
- Hypertriglyceridaemia
- Hepatic steatosis

SAQ 9 What do you mean by TPN? How is it delivered?

TPN means total perenteral nutrition, delivered by catheter inserted to peripheral veins, maneuvered to central venous system, i.e. peripherally inserted central venous catheter PICC line (for less than 2 weeks time) or through central venous line (subclavian, internal jugular, etc. secreened by radiological guidance). It should be managed by dedicated team of specialist to avoid infection.

9 Burn

LAQ 1 Name the different types of thermal injuries.

THERMAL INJURIES

- **Due to cold**
  - **Local**
    - Frost bite
    - Trench foot
  - **General**
    - Hypothermia
- **Due to heat**
  - **Local**
    - Burn
    - Scald
  - **General**
    - Heat stroke
    - Heat cramps
    - Heat exhaustion

SAQ 2 What are the different types of burn injuries?

(i) Burns due to dry heat

(ii) Burns due to moist heat called **scalds**

(iii) Electric burn at point of entry and exit

(iv) Burns due to corrosive (acid or alkalis)

(v) Ionization radiation

SAQ 3 What are the factors which determine the prognosis of burn?

(i) Extent of burn (burn around face and neck and history of being trapped in burning room carries bad prognosis).

(ii) Severity of burn

(iii) Infection

LAQ 4 How the burns can be classified?

The different ways of classifying burns are:

Dupuytren's classification

1st degree
2nd degree
3rd degree
4th degree
5th degree
6th degree

Superficial or deep

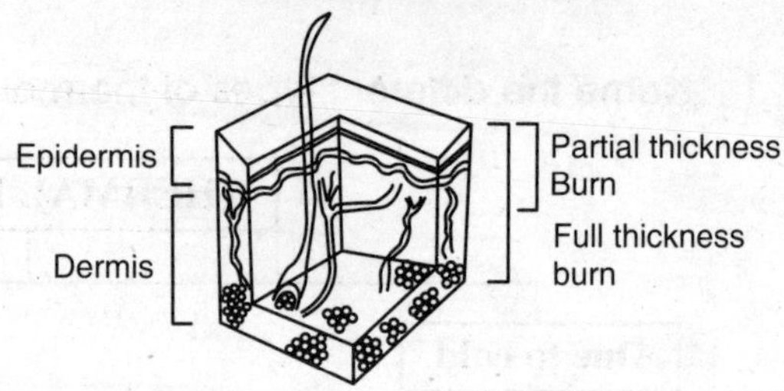

SAQ 5 What are the different ways of assessing burn wound?

The different methods are:

(i) **Wallace rule of nine**: Head and face 9%; upper limb (each) 9%; front of trunk 18%; back of trunk18%; lower limb each 18%; perineum 1%

(ii) **Land and Browder charts**

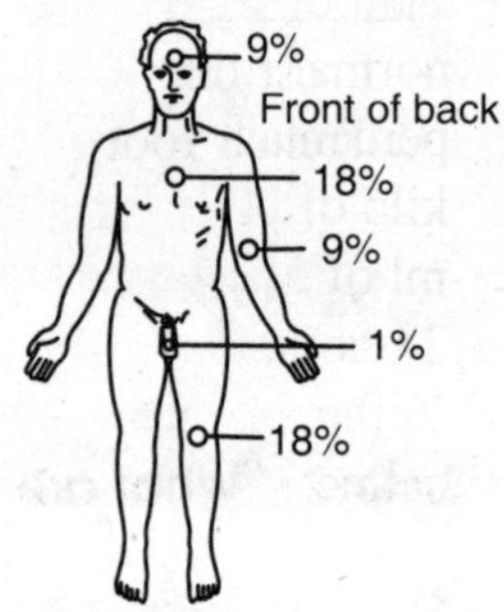

SAQ 6 What are the dangers of inhalation of smoke, gas, etc. in burn patient?

(i) Supraglottic burn and laryngeal oedema
(ii) Damage of respiratory epithelium and subglottic burn
(iii) Chemical alveolitis and respiratory failure
(iv) Mechanical blockage to respiration by burning of chest and ribs

LAQ 7 What is the principle of treatment of burn?

Burns should be treated keeping following things in mind:

(i) Local treatment
(ii) Treatment of shock
(iii) General treatment.

Treatment of shock

(i) Burnt area covered with sterile sheet

(ii) Morphine ¼ grain IV and repeated if required

(iii) Fluid replacement (children over 10% and adult over 15% requires IV fluid. Note urine output, salt to be added for oral fluids)

Calculation of fluids

Evan's formula

1 ml of plasma and 1 ml of normal saline for each percentage of burn per kilo of body weight +2000 ml of 5% dextrose in 1st 24 hours. In 2nd 24 hours, ½ the amount of plasma and saline + 2000 ml of 5% dextrose

Wallace formula

110 ml of plasma and 110 ml of normal saline for each 1% of burn in 48 hours divided into three rations in 0–8; 8–24; 24–48 hours

Parkland formula

Total percentage body surface × weight in kg × 4 = vol in ml given in ratio of two 8; 16 hours.

LAQ 8. How to care for local wound for burn?

The principle for local treatment of burn is as following:

Care of wound

(i) 1% silver sulfadiazine cream
(ii) 0.5% silver nitrate solution
(iii) Mafenide acetate cream
(iv) Serum nitrate

It may be done by exposure treatment or closed treatment

Splintage

Splintage is done for burns involving flexor surface of joints to prevent contracture

Skin grafting

The skin grafting is done for full thickness burn as early as possible or at 2 or 3 weeks

LAQ 9 How to manage post-burn contracture?

Prevention

- Splintage
- Treat and prevent infection
- Skin grafting

Treatment

- Z plasty
- Traction
- Full thickness grafts
- Pressure garments for hypertrophy
- Pharmacological treatment for itch

10 Warfare Injuries

SAQ 1 How the injuries caused by missile wounds are described?

They are now described as energy transfer not by velocities.

SAQ 2 How the low energy transfer wounds differ from high energy transfer wounds?

In low energy transfer wounds are confined to tracks but high energy transfer also causes wound remote to wound track called temporary cavitation. The cavity within solid organs such as kidney, liver or spleen increases mortality and morbidity. The cavity of devitalized muscles produces culture medium and that of bone may produce secondary missiles.

SAQ 3 What are the principles of treatment of missile injuries?

- Skin should be preserved but fascia should be divided
- Wound should leave open
- Remove devitalized tissues
- Vessels and nerves should be repaired
- Joints should be cleaned
- Bone should be stabilized and joint cavities should be closed
- Foreign matter should be removed

SAQ 4 How to recognize devitalized muscles?

The dead muscles:

- Do not bleed or contract
- Mushy in consistency without capillary bleeding.

SAQ 5 What are the principles of treatment of liver, spleen, pancreas, kidney, colon, injury by missiles?

Spleen: Resection or splenorrhaphy
Pancreas: Resection or Roux loop jejunum
Kidney: Try conservatively or rarely by nephrectomy

Colon: Primary repair or resection. Pelvic injuries may require ligature of internal iliac artery

Peritoneum: Peritoneal toilet with warm saline to remove spilled bowel and blood clots

SAQ 6 Mention the principle of missiles wound of the chest.

(i) Airtight seal to prevent pneumothorax followed by thoracostomy otherwise there will be collapse of lungs, dyspnoea, anoxia, mediastinal shifting, decrease venous return of heart
(ii) Venting of pleura is treated by formal tube thoracostomy
(iii) Foreign body should be removed
(iv) Closure of pleura by direct closure or by healthy soft tissue
(v) **Thoracotomy is required if:**
 (a) More than 1.5 blood loss; or loss more than 200 ml/hour continuously
 (b) Cardiac temponade
 (c) Injuries to mediastinal structure or air leakage or foreign body in pleura

SAQ 7 Which injuries are greater water, air by blast in?

Injury at water is greater, it may produce water hammer with significant effect, GI perforation.

SAQ 8 Which organs are primarily affected by blast injuries?

Primarily, it involves middle ear, lung and bowel.

SAQ 9 What is post-blast respiratory insufficiency (PBRI)?

The syndrome of PBRI resembles ARDS due to sepsis and fat embolism; which may be further aggravated by over transfusion.

SAQ 10 Mention the principle of treatment of PBRI.

- Post-blast respiratory insufficiency is treated with **advanced trauma life support (ATLS)**
- Avoid over infusion or transfusion
- Oxygen inhalation and perform arterial blood analysis
- Mechanical ventilation
- Avoid corticosteroids

11 Anaesthesia

SAQ 1 Who first demonstrated ether as anaesthesia?

John Colins Warren of Massachisetts General Hospital. WTG. Morton administered ether for dental extraction in 1846.

SAQ 2 What an anaesthetic provide during operation?

General anesthetics provide:

- Unconsciousness
- Pain relief
- Muscle relaxations

SAQ 3 What are the duties of an anaesthetist?

- Patient's safety and welfare
- Preoperative check up
- Optimise operating conditions and prevent injury
- Functions of preoperative physician

LAQ 4 What preoperative checks and investigations are must by an anaesthetist?

Preoperative check:

(i) **Cardiorespiratory system:** RTI, asthma, hypertension, ischaemia, arrhythmia, failure
(ii) **Metabolic:** Diabetes, steroid, porphyria
(iii) **Blood:** Haemoglobin, coagulation defects
(iv) **Neuro:** Psychiatric: consciousness, drugs
(v) **GIT:** Jaundice, bowel obstruction, etc.

Preoperative investigations

• TBC • Na; K • CXR(PA) • ECG. • Hepatitis B antigen • Blood group and gas tension

> Anaesthetist must take informed consent before operation for inducing anaesthesia

LAQ 5 Name the different drugs given before anaesthesia.

Preoperative

(i) **Sedative:** Analgesics, antitussives
(ii) **Anticholinergics** (glycopyrronium, atropine or hyoscine to reduce GI and respiratory secretions and vagal arrhythmia
(iii) **Antithrombotic** (subcutaneous heparin)
(iv) **Contraceptive** should be stopped
(v) **Antibiotic prophylactically**
(vi) **Bronchodilator** or physiotherapy

SAQ 6 What are the different methods of managing airway during anaesthesia?

(i) Thrust the jaw forward from behind, i.e. positioning the tongue and jaw.
(ii) Laryngeal mask airway
(iii) Endotracheal tube
(iv) Tracheostomy tube
(v) Endobronchial tube
(vi) Ventilation through bronchoscope.

SAQ 7 What complications may arise due to endotracheal tube?

- Accidental intubation into oesophagus or bronchus
- Trauma of tooth, trachea, larynx
- Aspiration, vomiting
- Blockage of tube
- Prolong intubation may produce stenosis

LAQ 8 What parameters should be monitored during anaesthesia?

- Inspiratory oxygen concentration
- Oxygen saturation by pulse oximetry
- Expiratory CO_2
- BP and ECG
- Ventilatory disconnection alarm
- Urinary output and renal perfusion
- Temperature measurement
- Neuromuscular monitoring if available.

LAQ 9 What are the causes of failure to breath after anaesthesia?

- Excessive sedation or opioid drugs
- Airways obstruction
- Hypoxia or hypercarbia
- Pneumothorax; circulatory failure
- Respiratory arrest
- Neuromuscular blockage

SAQ 10 What are the different techniques of local anaesthesia?

It may be:

- Infiltration
- Topical
- Field block
- Plexus block
- Intravenous block
- Epidural block
- Intrathecal block

SAQ 11 Name some local anaesthetics.

- Lignocaine
- Bupivacaine
- Ropivacaine
- Prilocaine

LAQ 12 How to manage postoperative pain?

1st — Paracetamol

↓

If no response then — NSAID

↓

If no response then — Codeine phosphate

↓

If no response then — Morphine

↓

If no response — Local anaesthesia (spinal; epidural)

↓

If no response then — Continuous epidural anaesthesia

or continuous IV or S/C infusion of anaesthesia

LAQ 13 Mention some of the neurolytic techniques in cancer pain.

In case of established diagnosis of cancer with limited life expectancy, following methods may be tried:

(i) Injection of phenol subcostally for ribs metastasis
(ii) Coeliac plexus neurolytic block
(iii) Hyperbaric injection of phenol intrathecally
(iv) Percutaneous anterolateral cordotomy to devide spinothalamic tract

Pharmacological methods

(i) Antipituitary hormone: Tamoxifen, cyproterone
(ii) Radiotherapy
(iii) Corticosteroids to reduce edema. Tricyclic antidepressants, anticonvulsants, etc.

12 Principles of Oncology

SAQ 1 What is carcinogens?

Agents that cause cancer are called ***carcinogens***. It may be initiator or promoter of cancers, e.g. polycyclic hydrocarbon groups or others like physical, chemical or infective agents.

SAQ 2 What do you mean by oncogenes and tumour suppressor genes?

Oncogenes disrupt the regulation of intracellular pathways. Tumorigenesis is multistep process with multiple genetic mutation. Oncogenes function as growth factor or tyrosine kinase.

On the other hand, **tumour suppressor genes** (TSG) inactivate tumourigenesis. Tumour suppressor genes may be functionally losed by mutation, deletions, protein phosphorylation.

SAQ 3 What is apoptosis?

This physiological process with multiple steps with condensation and fragmentation of chromatin, shrinkage of cells which is taken up by macrophages without inflammatory reaction. It is dependent on induction of appropriate genes. Cancer cells are resistant to apoptosis.

SAQ 4 What are the stages of cell growth and division?

The five stages of cell growth and divisions are $G_{1;}$ S; $G_{2;}$ M and Go. Cyclins and cyclin-dependent kinases regulate cell cycles.

LAQ 5 What do you mean by Gemopertzian pattern of cell growth?

It means small tumours grow rapidly, but larger tumour growing slowly. The reason may be:

(i) Blood supply
(ii) Nutrition
(iii) Large growth fractions.

This may be the reason of susceptibility of small tumours for chemo- and radiotherapy.

LAQ 6 What are the causes of metastasis?

- Loss of cell to cell adhesion
- Proteolytic enzymes and
- Metalloproteinases responsible for cellular metastasis with some organ specificity.

Dissemination of tumour cells may occur through:

- Blood
- Lymphatics
- Coelomic spaces

SAQ 7 What do you mean by TNM system of classification?

The extent of spread of primary tumour (T), spread to local lymph node (N) and presence of metastasis (M) is accepted system for tumour classification by Union Internationale Contre le Cancer (UICC).

M_0 = Without metastasis; M_1 = Metastasis; Mx-Not possible to determine metastasis.

SAQ 8 What do you mean by screening of cancer?

Screening of cancers means detecting asymptomatic cancers. It provides early diagnosis and to prevent morbidity and mortility treatment. The screening test should be safe, inexpensive, acceptable and sensitive.

SAQ 9 What are the different approaches of cancer treatment?

It is done by multidisciplinary team and different methods are: (i) surgery, (ii) chemotherapy, (iii) Radiotherapy.

SAQ 10 How surgery helps treatment of cancer?

It is used to:

- Diagnose
- Remove primary and distant metastasis
- Palliation
- Prevention and
- Reconstruction.

LAQ 11 What is the mechanism of action of radiotherapy?

Directly

By interacting with tissues

Indirectly

Produces reactive species by breaking down water which damages macromolecules.

SAQ 12 What are the factors which determine effect of radiotherapy?

(i) Sensitivity
(ii) Size of tumours
(iii) Site of tumours

LAQ 13 What are the complications of radiotherapy?

(i) Bone marrow suppression
(ii) Gonads suppression
(iii) Cataract
(iv) Nausea vomiting, diarrhoea, mucositis
(v) Erythema
(vi) Brown-Séquard's syndrome
(vii) Pneumonitis
(viii) Nephritis
(ix) Liver failure
(x) Stunted growth
(xi) Cancer

SAQ 14 What do you mean by GTV; CTV; PTV?

GTV: Gross tumour volume
CTV: Clinical target volume (also includes undetectable tumour cells)
PTV: Planning target volume

SAQ 15 What are the different types of chemotherapeutic agents for cancer cells?

It can be grouped into:
(i) **Alkylating agents** (cyclophosphamide, melphalan, nitrogen mustard, etc.)
(ii) **Antimetabolite** (5 FU; methotrexate, 6MP; cytosine arabinoside, etc.)
(iii) **Vinca alkaloids:** (vincristine, vinblastine, vindesine, etc.)

(iv) **Antibiotics:** Adriamycin, bleomycin, actinomycin D, mitomycin, etc.
(v) **Miscellaneous**

SAQ 16 What are the other forms of therapy for cancer?

(i) **Hormone therapy**
(ii) **Immunotherapy** (levamesole, interferon, BCG)
(iii) **Gene therapy**
(iv) **Biological modifiers** (metalloproteinase inhibitors, epidermal growth factor antagonist)

Day Surgery, Surgical Audit and Statistics

13

LAQ 1 What do you mean by day surgery? What are its benefits and problems?

In day surgery, patient is admitted and discharged on the same day with planned investigation and procedures but require some time for recovery.

Its benefits are:

(i) Cheap with better use of resources
(ii) Time-saving for patient
(iii) Less cancellation of surgery
(iv) Complications are less
(v) Patients prefer it.

Problems:

(i) Risk of morbidity and mortility
(ii) Initial cost of set up
(iii) Care by family with less information.

SAQ 2 Which patients are suitable for day surgery?

(i) Where chances of blood loss are less
(ii) Postoperative complications are less
(iii) Less physiological challenge
(iv) Pain controllable with oral analgesics and patient can walk after operation.

LAQ 3 Which patient should not be booked for day surgery?

Patient with:

(i) **CVS diseases** (hypertension, angina, cardiomyopathy, valvular disease)
(ii) **Respiratory diseases:** Asthma, COPD.
(iii) **Miscellaneous:** Diabetic on insulin, alcoholic, neurological disease (myasthenia, narcotic addicts, spondylosis)
(iv) **On drugs:** Anticoagulant, MAO-1, digoxin, steroids, OCP, antiarrhythmic, etc.

SAQ 4 What are the guidelines for safe discharge after day surgery?

(i) Patient should not be vomiting, bleeding or with excessive pain
(ii) Patient should be oriented, take oral fluid, can dress, void and walk without assistance.

Patient should be discharged by surgeons and anaesthetist.

SAQ 5 What is audit cycle in surgery?

We rarely achieve perfection but by auditing we can strive towards perfection.
Stages are:

(i) Preparing audit
(ii) Selecting criteria
(iii) Measuring performance
(iv) Making improvements
(v) Keeping up improvements.

SAQ 6 What are the questions to be answered before understanding a research project?

Following things to be kept in mind before research is started.

(i) Necessity of the study
(ii) Whether the study is practical and answer the necessary questions and done with available resources.
(iii) The impact of study and expected findings

LAQ 7 Why it is necessary for statistical analysis?

As whole population cannot be included in studies, statistical analysis is required to see the difference between control and treated groups. The studies may be:

Observational

Conditions are compared

(i) Case control study
(ii) Cross-sectional
(iii) Longitudinal

Experimental

Treatments are compared

(i) Random study
(ii) Randomised control

SAQ 8 What do you mean by type I and type II errors?

Type I error
False +ve

Perceived benefit without reality

Type II error
False –ve

Missed benefit

SAQ 9 What is ethics?

The ethics is that, which has some moral values. Common sense is the best ethics. Ask ethical committee in case of doubts.

SAQ 10 What is SERNP?

Safety and **E**fficacy **R**egister of **N**ew intervention **P**rocedure used in the UK and Australia. They give permission for new therapeutic procedures.

SAQ 11 What do you mean by parametric and non-parametric tests?

In **parametric** test, normally distributed "t" test is used to compare treatment and control.

In **non-parametric** method, Chi-Square, Wilcoxon signed rank test or Mann-Whitney U test can be used.

SAQ 12 What is CONSORT?

It stands for Consolidated Standards of Report Trials, which guidelines conduct of clinical trials.

14 Basic Surgical Skills

SAQ 1 What precaution should be taken to suture a skin?

- It should be sutured with minimum tension
- Edges should be slightly gaping to allow swelling in the edges
- Edges should be everted
- Knots should be tight at the end and space should be there at a end to remove suture

SAQ 2 What are the different types of skin suture?

It may be: (i) Continuous or interrupted
(ii) Simple; mattress, subcuticular

SAQ 3 What are advantages of modern synthetic materials?

They are more completely absorbed, give predictable strength with minimal inflammatory reaction.

LAQ 4 Name some suture materials?

Some suture materials are following:

Non-absorbable

- Metal suture and clips (linear stapler, side to side stapler, end-to-end stapler)
- Silk
- Linen
- Surgical steel
- Nylon
- Polyester
- Polybutester
- Polypropylene

Absorbable

- Catgut (plain; chromic)
- Polyglactin
- Polyglyronate
- Polyglycolic acid
- Polydiaxanone
- Polyglycaprone

SAQ 5 Name the different types of knots.

It may be:

- Half hitch
- Reef
- Extra-half hitch on reef knot
- Crossed half hitch
- Granny
- Surgeon's knots

SAQ 6 What do you mean by anastomosis?

By anastomosis, tubular viscus (bowel) or vessels are joined after resection or bypass without exteriorisation with a stroma or having been tied off.

SAQ 7 What are the complications of vessel anastomosis?

- Leakage
- Bleeding
- Stenosis

15 Thyroid Gland

SAQ 1 How the thyroid gland is developed?

It develops from median bud of the pharynx (thyroglossal duct), passing from foramen caecum of tongue. Ultimo-bronchial body arising from 4th pharyngeal pouches of each side fuses to form lateral lobes. Parafollicular (C cells) arises from neural crest.

SAQ 2 What is the normal weight of thyroid gland?

20–25 gm

SAQ 3 Name the different hormones secreted from thyroid gland.

- Tri-iodothyronine (T_3)
- Thyroxine (T_4)
- Thyrocalcitonin

LAQ 4 Mention in brief the thyroid function tests.

Several tests are performed to assess the thyroid functions, because no single test is conclusive.

The assessment of thyroid functions can be done directly or indirectly as shown in the chart.

Thyroid function tests

Direct tests

1. Measurement of thyroid hormone (protein bound iodine; total and free serum T_4 and T_3
2. Measurement of free binding sites for thyroid hormones in the blood (in hyperthyroidism, it is low)
3. Uptake and discharge of ^{131}I by thyroid gland
4. T_3 suppression test of Werner
5. Thyroid scanning
6. Thyroid autoantibodies
7. FNAC

Indirect tests

1. BMR
2. ECG
3. Serum cholesterol
4. Tendon reflexes

Optional tests

- CXR (PA)
- USG
- CT
- MRI
- Calcium and albumin estimation
- Laryngoscope; truncut or large bone needle biopsy

SAQ 5 What is struma ovari?

It is ovarian teratoma containing thyroid tissue may produce hyperthyroidism or turn neoplastic.

SAQ 6 What are the peculiarities of thyroid swelling?

It moves with swallowing and/or on protruding the tongue.

SAQ 7 What is thyroglossal cyst?

It is remnant in thyroglossal tract, present anywhere in thryroglossal tract, but common sites are beneath the hyoid and above the hyoid bone.

A thyroglossal cyst more than 1 cm should be excised to prevent infection. Infected thyroglossal cyst if incised may produce fistula.

SAQ 8 What is cretinism and myxoedema?

Hypothyroid in infant is ***cretinism*** and that of adult is ***myxoedema***.

SAQ 9 What are the causes of hypothyroidism?

1. Autoimmune (nongoitrous) and goitrous (Hashimato's disease)
2. Iatrogenic (thyroidectomy; drug-induced or ^{131}I therapy)
3. Dyshormogenesis
4. Goitrogens
5. Diseases of hypothalamus and pituitary
6. Endemic iodine deficiencies
7. Agenesis of thyroid

LAQ 10 How a patient of hypothyroidism presents?

Clinical features of hypothyroidism

Symptoms

- Lethergy
- Tiredness
- Weight gain, cold intolerance
- Constipation
- Carpal tunnel syndrome
- Menstrual disturbances

Signs

- Bradycardia
- Cold extremities
- Dryness of skin and hair
- Periortrital puffiness
- Slow movement
- Delayed ankle jerk
- Midarosis

LAQ 11 What is goitre? What are their types?

It is enlargement of thyroid gland.

Types of goitre

- **Simple**
  - (Euthyroid)
  - Diffuse hyperplastic (Graves' disease)
  - Nodular
- **Toxic**
  - Toxic nodular
  - Diffuse toxic
  - Toxic nodule
- **Neoplastic**
  - Benign
  - Malignant
  - Riedel
- **Thyroiditis**
  - Granulomatous
  - Autoimmune
- **Rare goitre**
  - Amyloid
  - Acute and chronic bacterial thyroiditis

SAQ 12 What is goitrogens?

The substances producing goiter like:

- Vegetables (cabbage, kale, rape)
- Drugs (thyocynate, PAS, antithyroid drugs)

SAQ 13 What are the important complications of nodular goitre?

- Tracheal obstruction
- Secondary thyrotoxicosis
- Carcinoma

SAQ 14 How to treat simple goitre?

- Iodised table salt
- t-thyroxine

SAQ 15 How a retrosternal thyroid may present?

- Dyspnoea
- Cough,
- Stridor
- Dysphagia
- Engorged neck vein and superficial veins on chest
- Recurrent laryngeal nerve paralysis.

SAQ 16 What is thyroid incidentaloma?

These are clinically unsuspected and impalpable thyroid swelling, diagnosed during the use of image modalities for neck and non-thyroid head.

LAQ 17 What is thyrotoxicosis? What are its types?

It is hyperthyroid state but all its features are not due to raised thyroid hormones, so it as called thyrotoxicosis.

Types of thyrotoxicosis are:

(i) Graves' disease (diffuse toxic goitre)
(ii) Toxic nodular goitre
(iii) Toxic nodule
(iv) Miscellaneous causes

LAQ 18 How a patient of hyperthyroid presents?

Clinical features of hyperthyroidism

Symptoms

- Tiredness
- Emotional
- Heat intolerance
- Loss of weight
- Hunger increased
- Palpitation

Signs

- Hot and moist palm
- Tachycardia
- Exophthalmos
- Lid lag
- Goitre with bruits

SAQ 19 What are the eye signs of thyrotoxicosis?

- Exophthalmos
- Sclera can be seen on upper margin of cornea
- Conjunctival injection and chemosis
- Lid lag
- Oedema of eyelids

LAQ 20 What are the different types of treatment for thyrotoxicosis?

Antithyroid drugs

Disadvantage
- Prolong treatment

Advantage
- No surgery
- No radio-active substance

Surgery

Advantage
- High cure rate

Disadvantage
- Recurrence

Radio-iodine

Advantage
- No surgery,
- Short therapy

Disadvantage
- Availability

SAQ 21 What is (a) Thyrotoxicosis factitia, (b) Jod-Basedow thyrotoxicosis, (c) de Quervain's thyrotoxicosis?

Thyrotoxicosis factitia	Jod-Basedow thyrotoxicosis	de-Quervain's thyroiditis
Hyperthyroidism in patient taking thyroxin	Large doses of iodine given for hyperplastic endemic goitre causing thyrotoxicosis.	Mild hyperthyroidism due to autoimmune thyroiditis

SAQ 22 What postoperative complications may arise out of thyroidectomy?

(i) Haemorrhage and tension haematoma
(ii) Respiratory obstruction
(iii) Thyroid deficiency
(iv) Parathyroid deficiency
(v) Thyroid storm
(vi) Infection of wound
(vii) Keloid and hypertropic scar
(viii) Stich granuloma with or without sinus formation

LAQ 23 Classify thyroid neoplasm.

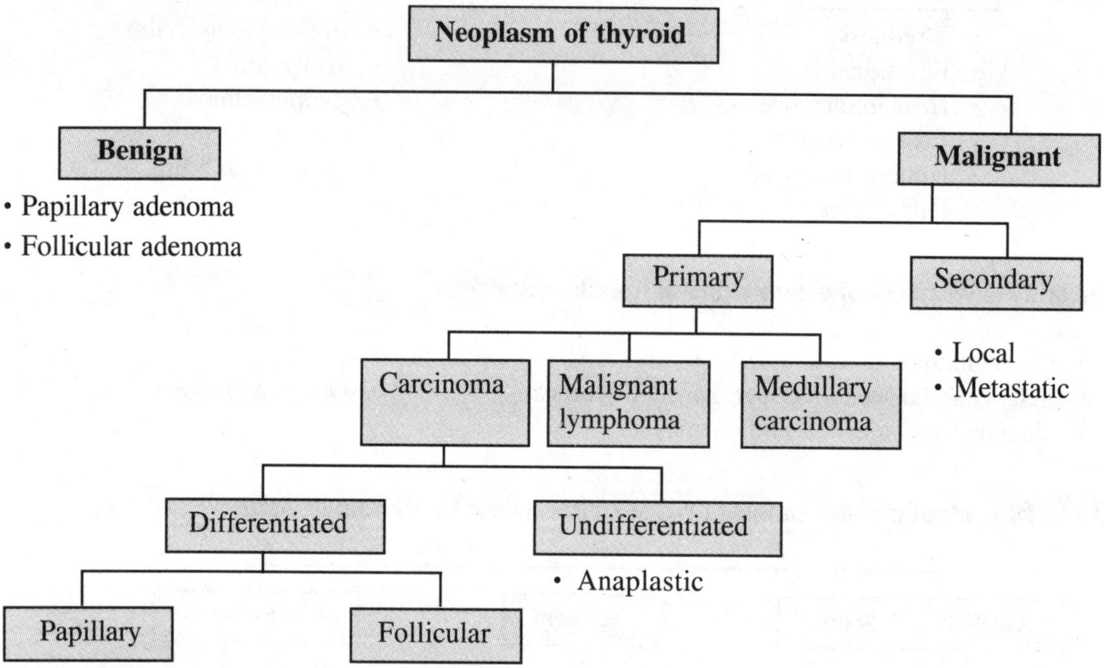

SAQ 24 What are the different types of thyroiditis?

These are:

(i) Chronic lymphocytic (autoimmunie) thyroiditis
(ii) Granulomatous thyroiditis (de Quervain's thyroiditis)
(iii) Riedel's thyroiditis

16 Parathyroid Gland

SAQ 1 What is the dimension and weight of parathyroid gland?

It is up to 6 mm in length and weighs up to 30–50 mg.

SAQ 2 How parathyroid glands are developed?

The superior parathyroid develops from 4th pharyngeal pouch and inferior from 3rd pharyngeal pouch.

SAQ 3 What is the function of parathyroid gland?

Parathyroid gland secretes 84 A. A containing parathormone,which on binding PTH receptor controls blood and extracellular calcium level.

SAQ 4 What is primary hyperparathyroidism?

Primary hyperparathyroidism occurs sporadically on familial with raised PTH and parathyroid enlargements.

LAQ 5 How a patient of hyperparathyroidism presents?

Bone: Pain, fracture, osteopenia

GIT: Peptic ulcer, pancreatitis, constipation

Kidney: Stone

Muscle: Fatigue

Soft tissue calcification

CVS: Hypertension, arrhythmia, calcification

Psychiatric: Dementia, anxiety

Others: Hyperuricaemia; insulin resistance, increased LDL and VLDL and low HDL.

LAQ 6 What are the different modes of treatment of hyperparathyroidism?

Medical

- Oestrogen supplement or bisphosphonate therapy
- Hydration
- Avoid calcium intake
- Calcium receptor antagonist

Surgical (indications)

- Urinary calculi
- Reduced bone density
- Raised serum calcium

SAQ 7 What is secondary hyperparathyroidism?

In case of low serum calcium as in CRF or malabsorption, there is secondary compensatory hypertrophy of parathyroid gland called secondary hyperparathyroidism, may require surgical treatment when bone pain and decalcification is severe.

SAQ 8 What are the causes of hypoparathyroidism?

(i) **Congenital**: Digeorge syndrome (thymic aplasia, absent parathyroid and cardiac defects); autoimmune polyglandular syndrome type I
(ii) **Acquired**: Wilson's disease, haemochromatosis, thyroidectomy

SAQ 9 What is Chvostek's sign and Trousseau's sign?

Thsese are signs of hypoparathyroidism:

Chvostek's sign	Trousseau's sign
Taping over branches of facial nerve will produce twitching of facial muscles	There will carpopedal spasm if sphygnomanometer cuff inflated above systolic BP

SAQ 10 How to treat tetany or hypoparathyroidism?

(i) IV calcium gluconate 10% (10–20 ml)
(ii) Oral vitamin D calciferol
(iii) Magnesium supplements.

17 Adrenal Gland

SAQ 1 How the adrenal gland develops?

Adrenal cortex is mesodermal in origin. ***Adrenal medulla*** dcvclops from neural crest cells.

SAQ 2 What are the layers of adrenal cortex?

It has three layers: (1) zona glomerulosa, (2) zona fasciculata and (3) zona reticularis secreting mineralocorticoids, glucocorticoids and sex hormones, respectively.

SAQ 3 Mention the different tests for adrenal cortical activity.

(i) Estimation of 24 hours output of urinary cortisol measurement
(ii) Estimation of plasma cortisol (8–28 μg/dl normal)
(iii) ACTH stimulation tests
(iv) Adrenal suppression test with cortisol or dexamethasone.
(v) Morphology of the gland is assessed by CT or MRI.

SAQ 4 What is Conn's syndrome?

Primary hyperaldosteronism due to unilateral adrenocortical adenoma.

SAQ 5 What are the causes of primary hyperaldosteronism?

(i) Conn's syndrome
(ii) Glucocorticoid suppressible hyeraldosteronism
(iii) Multiple adenoma
(iv) Unilateral hyperplasia
(v) Malignant aldosteronoma.

LAQ 6 What is Addison's disease? How it presents and treated?

It is chronic insufficiency of adrenocortical function.

It presents:

- Weight loss
- Skin and mucosal hyperpigmentation
- Hypotension
- Hyponatraemia
- Hyperkalaemia
- Low plasma cortisol and high basal ACTH.
- Treated with oral hydrocortisone, fluorocortisone.

SAQ 7 What is Waterhouse-Friderichsen syndrome?

It is an acute condition producing bilateral adrenal infraction, caused by haemorrhage, or sepsis (by meningococcal or *Pseudomonas*). It is highly fatal, if not treated properly.

SAQ 8 What is Cushing's syndrome?

It is a condition due to excess circulating cortisol (either ACTH dependent or ACTH independent)

LAQ 9 What are the clinical features of Cushing's syndrome?

It may present with:

- Weight gain
- Muscle weakness
- Hirsutism
- Pigmentation of skin
- Tiredness
- Thirst
- Renal stone
- Glucose intolerance
- Abdominal striae
- Acne
- Easy bruising
- Menstrual irregularities in female
- Impotence
- Headache
- Back pain due to osteoporosis and fracture

SAQ 10 How is Cushing's syndrome treated?

- Medically by metyrapone or ketoconazole
- Trans-sphenoidal excision of pituitary dependent microadenoma
- Radiotherapy
- Bilateral adrenalectomy (patient undergone adrenalectomy should be given postoperative steroids).

SAQ 11 What is incidentaloma?

It is incidentally discovered adrenal mass.

SAQ 12 What is adrenogenital syndrome?

It is an autosomal recessive disorder producing excess of adrenal androgens.

SAQ 13 Name the sites from where adrenal matastasis can take place.

- Breast
- Lung
- Kidney
- Melanoma
- Lymphoma.

LAQ 14 What is adrenal paraganglioma or phaeochromocytoma?

Adrenal paraganglioma or phaeochromocytoma is catecholamine producing turmour derived from chromaffin cells of adrenal medulla.
Other sites of paraganglioma:

(i) Abdominal para-aortic
(ii) Thorax
(iii) Bladder
(iv) Rarely neck and pelvis

LAQ 15 How a patient of pheochromocytoma presents?

- Intermittent hypertension
- Headache
- Weight loss
- Weakness
- Anxiety
- Bending straining or lifting may precipitate the attack.
- Paroxysm of sweating
- Palpitation lasting minutes to hours
- Pallor
- Visual disturbances
- Arrhythmia.

LAQ 16 How to treat phaeochromocytoma?

(i) With α blockers (phenoxybenzamine or doxazosin)
(ii) Surgery by skilled surgeon and anaesthetist
(iii) Malignant pheochromocytoma is treated with: (a) α blockers, (b) surgery, (c) combination of vincristine, dacarbazine and cyclophosphamide
(iv) Phaeochromocytoma with pregnancy treated with α blocker, caesarean section in third trimester.

SAQ 17 How to diagnose phaeochromocytoma?

(i) Estimation of VMA
(ii) Clonidine suppression test
(iii) It is better to avoid provocation tests.
(iv) Tumour is localized by CT/MRI and ^{123}I MIBG (metaiodobenzylguanidine)

SAQ 18 What is neuroblastoma? How is it treated?

This is malignant adrenal tumour derived from undifferentiated cells of sympathetic nervous system, often associated with catecholamine production. It may arise from neuroblast of extra-adrenal sites, viz. mediastinum, retroperitoneal.

It is treated with cyclophosphamide, cisplastin, doxorubicin followed by surgery and adjuvant radiotherapy.

SAQ 19 What is ganglioneuroma?

The ganglioneuroma is benign tumour with ganglion cells, Schwann cells and collagens of sympathetic nervous system, treated by surgical excision.

SAQ 20 Name some conditions when bilateral adrenalectomy done when disease is not there.

For inoperable breast or prostate carcinoma or their metastasis.

SAQ 21 Name some hereditary syndrome with which pheochromocytoma may occur.

- Multiple endocrine neoplasia 2A (Sipple syndrome)
- von Hippel-Lindau disease
- von Recklinghausen's disease or neurofibromatosis type I.

18 Liver

LAQ 1 What are the functions of liver?

Functions of liver are:

(i) Secretion of bile and haemoglobin degradation
(ii) Maintaining body temperature, pH and correction of lactic acidosis
(iii) Production of fibrinogen, prothrombin and albumin
(iv) Formation of cholesterol, and fatty acids from carbohydrate
(v) Deamination of amino acid and formation of urea
(vi) Removal of gut endotoxins and exoallergens
(vii) Storage of vitamin A, B_{12}, Fe and Cu
(viii) Metabolism of drugs and hormones
(ix) Destruction of bacteria
(x) Glucose metabolism
(xi) Reticulo-endothelial activities.

SAQ 2 What is the peculiarity of blood supply of liver?

Eighty per cent of its blood supply is from portal vein and twenty per cent from hepatic artery.

LAQ 3 Mention the important tests for liver.

(i) Estimation of: (a) bilirubin, (b) alkaline phosphatase, (c) aspartate transaminase, (d) gamma glutamyl transpeptidase, (e) albumin, (f) prothrombin time
(ii) Bromosulphalein test
(iii) Scanning of liver with colloidal gold 198 or technetium 99m
(iv) Ultrasonography
(v) Liver biopsy by Menghini needle
(vi) Arteriography by coeliac axis or superior mesenteric arteriogram
(vii) Computer X-ray scanning
(viii) CT, MRI, ERCP
(ix) Percutaneous transhepatic cholangiography (PTC)
(x) Laparoscopy and laparoscopic ultrasound

LAQ 4 What are causes of hepatomegaly?

Hepatomegaly

- Generalized
  - With jaundice
    - Viral hepatitis
    - Cholangitis
    - Pyelophlebitis
    - Ca pancreatic head
    - Ca CBD
    - Secondary deposit
  - Without jaundice
    - Cirrhosis
    - Budd-Chiari syndrome
    - CCF
    - Amyloid
    - Leukemia
- Irregular
  - Secondary
  - Gumma
- Localized
  - Riedal lobe
  - Amoebic hepatitis
  - Hydatid cyst

SAQ 5 What is intermittent fever of Charcot?

In cholangitis or intermittent hepatic fever of Charcot, inflammation of the biliary tree within the liver takes place. Etiologies are:

- Gallstone
- Suppurative cholangitis
- Stricture
- Pyelophlebitis
- Mucoviscidosis

It may be followed by formation of multiple liver abscess

SAQ 6 What is portal pyaemia?

Portal pyaemia or pyelophlebitis can occur due to suppuration in any part being drained by portal vein, viz. appendicitis.

LAQ 7 What are the causes of abscesses in liver?

The abscess of liver may enroute through:

1. Portal vein (appendicitis, diverticulitis, amoebiasis, ulcerative colitis, typhoid, inflamed piles)
2. Via bile duct (stone or stricture of CBD)
3. Hepatic artery (septicemia)
4. Via umbilicus
5. From adjacent structure (empyema thoracis, penetrating wound, subdiaphragmatic abscess)

SAQ 8 What is Caroli's disease?

Caroli's disease is congenital dilatation of intrahepatic biliary tree, may be complicated by stone formation, presents with pain abdomen and sepsis.

SAQ 9 How the amoebic liver abscess presents?

Amoebic liver presents as following:

- Anaemia
- Weight loss
- Earthly complexion
- Fever with rigor and sweating
- Pain right hypochondrium with enlargement and tenderness
- Basal lung signs.

LAQ 10 What are the indications, contraindications and complications of liver transplantation?

Liver transplantation

Indications

- Cirrhosis (diuretic resistant, encephalopathy, portal hypertension, hepatorenal failure)
- Primary biliary cirrhosis
- Alcoholic hepatitis
- Chronic HCV infection
- Sclerosing cholangitis

Contraindications

- Cholangio Ca
- Uncontrolled sepsis
- Widespread malignancy
- Cardiopulmonary disease

Complications

- Graft rejection
- Opportunistic infection
- Recurrent liver diseases

SAQ 11 What is honeycomb liver?

Honeycomb liver is fungal infection of liver by *Actinomyces israeli* entering liver by portal vein, hepatic artery or contiguous spread. Treated by exploration and long acting penicillin and other antibiotics.

SAQ 12 What is Budd-Chiari syndrome?

It is obstructions of hepatic veins. Presents with nausea, vomiting, pain in liver or death.

LAQ 13 Name the different neoplasms of liver.

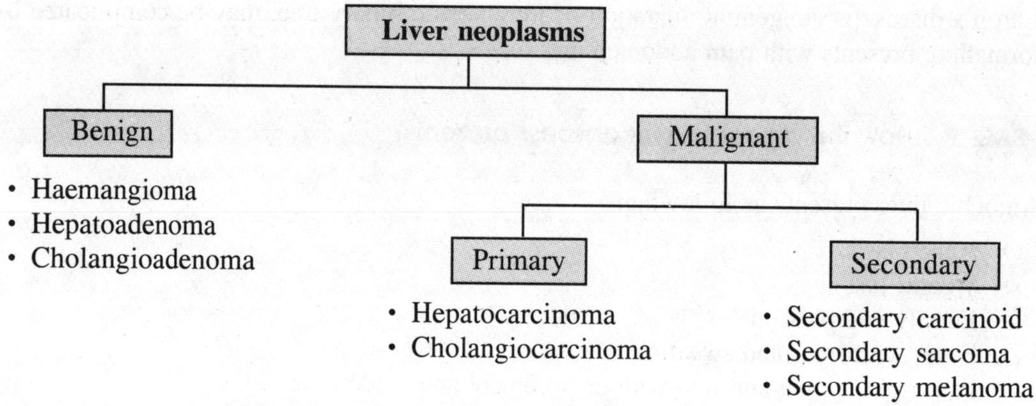

SAQ 14 How to treat oesophageal varices?

(i) Blood transfusion
(ii) Balloon temponade by Sengstaken-Blakemore tube
(iii) Drugs vasopressin/octreotide
(iv) Sclerosing or bonding
(v) TIPSS (transjugular intrahepatic portosystemic stent shunts)
(vi) Surgery (portosystemic shunting; oesophageal transaction; splenectomy and gastric devascularisation)

SAQ 15 What is portal hypertension are Froid?

It is portal hypertension but not bleeding dangerously or frankly.

SAQ 16 What are the different types of portosystemic operation?

(i) End-to-side portocaval anastomosis
(ii) Side-to-side portocaval anastomosis
(iii) Splenorenal anastomosis
(iv) Mesentericocaval anastomosis
(v) Mesentericorenal H graft
(vi) Distal splenorenal shunts.

SAQ 17 What is TIPSS?

It is stands for transjugular intrahepatic portosystemic stent shunts.

19 Spleen

SAQ 1 How the spleen develops?

It develops from condensation of mesoderm in dorsal mesogastrium.

LAQ 2 Describe in brief the anatomy of spleen.

Weighing 75–250 gm in left hypochondrium and left hemidiaphragm, long axis on 10th rib, supplied by tortuous splenic artery. Splenic vein is formed by several tributaries, joins superior mesenteric vein to form portal vein.

Lymphatic – efferent vessels from white pulp from nodes in hilum and through retropancreatic nodes drain coeliac nodes.

Sympathetic innervation from coeliac plexus innervate splenic arterial branches.

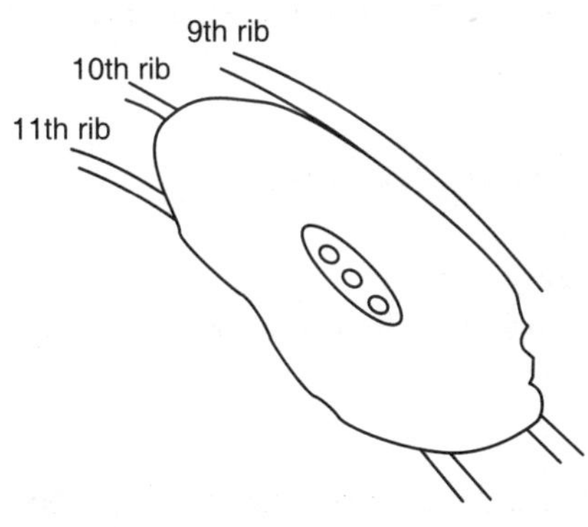

Spleen

LAQ 3 What are the functions of the spleen?

- **Immune function:** Specific: produce IgM
  Non-specific: Produce oppsonin, properdin, tuftsin.
- **Filter function:** Macrophages of reticulum engulf cellular and noncellular materials from blood and plasma.
- **Pitting:** Particulate materials from RBC are removed.

- **Erythropoiesis and cytopoiesis:** Produce RBC, produce T and B cells, macrophages
- **Reservoir of RBC**
- **Hormone regulation of the marrow:** Which inhibits production of thrombocytes and leukocytes.

SAQ 4 What is splenunculi and splenosis?

Splenunculi is accessory spleen.

Splenosis is fragments of spleen spilled on peritoneum.

SAQ 5 What are different special investigations for spleen?

- Radiography (plain X-ray, CT, MRI, technetium 99m lebelled to determine whether it is significant site of RBC destruction)
- Splenic puncture
- Splenopartography

SAQ 6 Mention some congenital abnormalities of spleen.

• Splenunculi • Splenosis • Splenic agenesis • Wandering or movable spleen • Torsion of splenic pedicle.

SAQ 7 How to treat splenic artery aneurysm?

Splenectomy and removal of diseased artery.

If it is not possible to excise, it should be ligated at proximal and distal ends to allows thrombosis of the aneurysm.

LAQ 8 What are the important causes of splenic infarction?

- Splenomegaly due to myeloproliferative syndrome
- Portal hypertension
- Vascular occlusion by pancreatic disease
- Splenic vein thrombosis
- Sickle cell disease

Treatement

Diagnosed by contrast-enhanced CT showing perfusion defects.

Treated conservatively or splenectomy, if septic infarct producing abscess.

SAQ 9 What are the different modes of presentations for splenic rupture?

Splenic rupture is dangerous event, may present as:

1. Patients succumbs from huge haemorrhage and never rallying from shock
2. Initial shock, temponade, signs of late bleeding and ruptured spleen
3. Delayed type of case when catastrophe are postponed up to 15 days or more

SAQ 10 What are the signs of rupture spleen?

Signs of haemorrhage: Pallor, tachycardia, sigh respiration, restlessness

Local signs:

- Abdominal rigidity,
- Tenderness,
- Balance sign (i.e. dull note on left side which is constant)
- Abdominal distension
- Kehr's sign positive (pain and hyperaesthesia of left shoulder)
- Rectal examination reveals tenderness and soft swelling of blood or clot.

SAQ 11 How to treat splenic rupture?

Laparotomy if possible, spleen should be preserved. Evacuate blood, minor capsular parenchymal injuries treated by local haemostat or partial segmental resection. Huge splenic rupture is treated by splenectomy. Rupture of malarial spleen is treated by splenectomy.

SAQ 12 What is autotransfusion?

Collection of extravasated blood from peritoneal cavity mixing it with 3.8%; Na-citrate and transfusing it IV.

LAQ 13 What postoperative complications may arise out of splenectomy?

- Haematemesis
- Acute dilatation of stomach
- Paralytic ileus
- Hiccough (peritoneal effusion)
- Pancreatic fistula
- Haemorrhage
- Left basal atelectasis
- Rheumatism
- Pancreatitis
- Opportunistic postsplenectomy infection.

SAQ 14 What is Felty's syndrome?

Felty's syndrome consists of following:

- Rheumatoid arthritis
- Leukopenia
- Splenic enlargement constitutes Felty's syndrome

LAQ 15 What are the causes of splenomegaly?

Splenomegaly

Infective causes	Blood disease	Metabolic causes	Circulatory causes	Miscellaneous
Bacterial: • Typhoid • Septicaemia • Syphilis • Weil's disease • Tb **Viral:** • HIV • Infectous mononucleosis **Parasite:** • Malaria • Kala-azar • Hydatid cyst	• ALL • CLL • Erythroblastosis • Polycythaemia	• Ricket • Amyloid • Porphyria • Goucher's disease	• Infarct • Portal hyper-tension	**Collagen:** Felty's and Still's disease **Neoplastic:** • Angioma • Fibrosarcoma • Hodgkin • Myelofibrosis

20 Gallbladder and Bile Duct

LAQ 1 Describe in brief the anatomy of gallbladder and bile duct.

Gallbladder develops from ventral wall of fore gut as hepatic diverticulum, stalk elongates to form choledochus.

It is pear-shaped, capacity 50 ml, parts are **infundibulum, neck, body and fundus**. Neck may be angulated to form Hartmann pouch. Mucosa sinks to muscle coat forming crypts of Luschka.

Left and right hepatic ducts combine to form common hepatic duct which joins to cystic duct and produce common bile duct (7.5 cm long). The common bile duct has four parts (supraduodenal, retroduodenal, infraduodenal, intraduodenal). Arterial supply is by cystic artery (branch of right hepatic artery). Lymphatics drain to cystic lymph node of Lund.

SAQ 2 What is Callot's triangle?

The arbitrary triangle whose three arms are produced by cystic duct and common hepatic duct and cystic artery.

SAQ 3 Mention the important functions of gallbladder.

It stores and concentrates bile. It secretes mucus also.

LAQ 4 Mention the important investigations of biliary tract.

- Plain radiograph
- USG
- Oral cholecystography
- Intravenous cholangiography
- Radioisotope scanner
- Magnetic resonance cholangiopancreatography (MRCP)
- Endoscopic retrograde cholangiopancreatography (ERCP)
- Percutaneous transhepatic cholangiography (PTC)
- Preoperative cholangiography
- Operative biliary endoscopy

SAQ 5 What are the different types of extrahepatic biliary atresia?

Type I : Atresia of CBD
Type II : Atresia of CHD
Type III : Atresia of right and left hepatic ducts

SAQ 6 How a patient of biliary atresia presents and treated?

Progressive jaundice at birth, bile stained meconium, pruritus, clubbing, xanthoma, pale stool

Type I: Lesion is treated by Roux-en-Y anastomosis

Type II and Type III: are treated by Kasai procedure where bile duct are excised up to liver capsule and Roux-en-Y of jejunum is anastomosed to exposed area of liver capsule above bifurcation of portal vein.

LAQ 7 What is choledochal cyst? How is it diagnosed and treated?

It is dilatation of common bile duct due to weakness of specific part or whole of CBD. It may be of following types:

Type I — Ia: Cysitc dilatation of particular portion
— Ib: Dilatation of whole CBD
Type II: Diverticulum of CBD
Type III: Diverticulum in pancreas
Type IV: Extension into the liver
Type V: Cystic dilation of intrahepatic duct

Diagnosed by USG and MRI

Treated by: Radical excision of the cyst with construction of biliary tract with Roux-en-Y loop of jejunum.

SAQ 8 How will you treat trauma of gallbladder?

Cholecystectomy and if there is involvement of CBD Roux-en-Y, choledochojejunostomy.

SAQ 9 What is cholesterosis or strawberry or fish scale gallbladder?

In this condition, cholesterol crystals are deposited in the mucus membrane of the gallbladder. Patient is advised low fat diet and cholagogues if there is no other pathology.

SAQ 10 What is Marcedes Benz or Seagul sign?

Here centre of the gallstone contains radiolucent gas in triradiate or biradiate fissure with dark shape on radiograph called Marcedes Benz or Seagul sign.

SAQ 11 What is Limey bile?

In this condition, gallbladder is filled with toothpaste like mixture of $CaCO_3$; $CaPO_4$, occurring if there is gradual obstruction of CBD; or cystic duct as in chronic pancreatitis or Ca pancreas. It is generally sterile and visualized in plain radiograph.

LAQ 12 What are the different types of gallstones?

GALLSTONES

- **Metabolic**
  - **Cholesterol stone**
    - Generally single (cholesterol solitaire)
    - Contains large cholesterol content in bile.
  - **Pigment stone**
    - **Brown pigment**
      - Contains Ca bilirubinate Ca palmitate, Ca stearate and cholesterol
      - Generally in bile duct
    - **Black pigment**
      - Insoluble bilirubin pigment with $CaPO_4$ and $CaCO_3$
      - Occurs in haemolytic condition or mechanical prosthesis
- **Infective or mixed**
  - Over the infection (evidenced by dead bacteria, RBC,WBC) alternate layer of bilirubin; $CaCO_3$ and cholesterol are deposited
  - Stones are moderate sized; multiple

SAQ 13 What are the predisposition factors of gallstone formation?

- Infection
- Bile stasis
- Hypercholesteremia

LAQ 14 Mention the important complications of gallstons.

In gallbladder: Chronic cholescystitis, mucocele, empyema, perforation, gangrene, carcinoma, calcification

In CBD: Jaundice, cholangitis

In pancreas: Pancreatitis

In intestine: Paralytic gallstone ileus.

LAQ 15 How a gallstone patient presents?

No symptoms or dyspepsia, epigastric or subcostal pain (Rt) generally at night may radiate to shoulder. It may resolve or may become systematically unwell. Fever, vomiting, upper abdominal guarding (Murphy's sign), jaundice, cholangitis or other features of gallstone complications may occur.

SAQ 16 What is Murphy's sign?

There will be catch of respiration if inflamed gallbladder if palpated. When it is done by patient lying it is called Moynihan's sign.

LAQ 17 Write short notes on stones in the CBD.

CBD stones are mostly secondary gallstones, usually pigment stone or mixed stones.

Effect of impacted stones:

- Obstructive jaundice
- Hydrohepatosis
- Acute pancreatitis
- White bile
- Hepatic failure

SAQ 18 How to treat stones in GB and GBD?

Stone in gallbladder is treated by cholecystectomy or laparoscopic cholecystectomy and that in CBD by choledocholithotomy.

SAQ 19 What is Charcot's triad?

Stones in CBD producing:

- Recurrent biliary colic
- Fluctuating jaundice and
- Intermittent fever with rigor (cholangitis) is called 'Charcot's triad'.

SAQ 20 What is Couvorsier's law?

If in a patient of obstructive jaundice with palpable gallbladder, then cause of obstruction is not impacted duct stone it is usually Ca head of pancreas, because in CBD stone, GB is inelastic and fibrotic incapable of dilating, but in Ca pancrease biliary pressure rises unopposed.

SAQ 21 What are the causes of biliary stricture?

- Trauma
- Parasites
- Bile duct injury
- Idiopathic
- Radiotherapy
- Gastrectomy
- Stones
- Pancreatitis
- Liver resection, etc.
- Cholangitis
- Biliary atresia

SAQ 22 Name some parasitic infestations of gallbladder.

(i) Biliary ascariasis (*Ascaris lumbricoides*)
(ii) Clonorchiasis by flukes
(iii) Hydatid cyst of gallbladder

SAQ 23 What is papillomatosis of gallbladder?

It is multiple mucus secreting tumour of biliary epithelium (low grade papillary carcinoma) treated by choledochoscopy with obliteration of the papillary lesions.

SAQ 24 What is Boas sign?

Area of hyperesthesia between 9th and 11th ribs posteriorly on right side in acute cholecystitis is called Boas sign.

SAQ 25 What is white bile?

It occurs following obstruction of CBD or common hepatic duct when gallbladder is not functioning or absent. It contains mucus of ducts, cholesterol, bile salt. It is misnomer because is neither bile or white in colour.

LAQ 26 Enumerate the factors associated with gallstone formation.

(a) **Impaired gallbladder function:** For example, impairment of emptying, absorption and excretion of gallbladder.
(b) **Supersaturated bile** as in aged perosn, genetically determined, obesity, high fatty diet.
(c) **Nucleating factors for cholesterol:** For example, mucus infection and glycoprotein.
(d) **Impaired enterohepatic circulation:** Faecal flora, ileal resection, cholestryramine, bowel transit.

21 Pancreas

SAQ 1 What is the meaning of the word pancreas?

Greek *Pan* = All; *Kreas* = Flesh

SAQ 2 How is the pancreas developed?

Two pancreatic buds from dorsal and ventral mesoduodenum develop which fuse to from pancreas.

SAQ 3 What are the ducts of pancreas?

(i) Duct of Wirsung runs along whole length of pancreas towards head and
(ii) Accessory duct of Santorini drains parts of the head (present in 10% of persons)

LAQ 4 Mention the important physiological functions of the pancreas.

Pancreas secretes digestive enzymes, bicarbonate rich secretion, cholecystokinin (CCK or pancreozymin) released from duodenal mucosa in response to food, secretes the enzymes. Vagal stimulation increases volume. Protein is sysnthesized in pancreas. Proteolytic enzymes are in inactive form which prevent pancreatitis. Insulin and glucagon are secreted by pancreas, responsible for glucose haemostat.

SAQ 5 Mention the important investigations of pancreatic diseases.

Some investigations of pancreatic diseases are:

(i) Pancreatic function tests
(ii) Pancreatic enzymes in body fluids
(iii) USG; CT; MRI; ERCP
(iv) Plain X-ray abdomen; CXR(PA); PET

LAQ 6 What are the causes of raised serum amylase in plasma?

Cases of raised serum amylase are:
- Pancreatitis
- Mesenteric infarction
- Torsion abdominal viscus
- Kidney failure
- Upper GI perforation
- Retroperitoneal haematoma
- Macroamylasaemia

LAQ 7 What is NBT-PABA test and PLT test?

Here **nitroblue tetrazolium para-amino benzoic acid (NBT-PABA)** is administered orally and uninary PABA is measured. NBT-PABA is broken by pancreatic chymotrypsin.

In **pancreolauryl test (PLT),** the substrate is fluorescein esterified by two lauric acids, hydrolysed by pancreatitic aryl esterase, the fluorescein liberated in gut lumen, absorbed and excreted by kidneys.

The test is performed for exocrine inefficiency of pancreas.

Faecal elastase estimation can detect chronic pancreatitis.

LAQ 8 What is cystic fibrosis?

This is autosomal recessive disorder which may develp pancreatitis in late life. There is abnormal exocrine gland function. Malabsorption (pancreatic insufficiency), abnormal lung function and increased Na^+ and Cl^- in sweat. Diabetes mellitus may occur in later life. Meconium ileus, steatorrhoea, poor growth, distended abdomen, persistent cough, emphysema, clubbing may be the presenting features in children. Cirrhosis, portal hypertension, corpulmonale, delayed appearance of secondary sex character are other features.

Diagnosis is confirmed by high Na and Cl ions in sweat.

Treatment: low fat diet, enzyme supplements, physiotherapy and antibiotics, extra salt for its loss through sweat.

SAQ 9 What is annular pancreas?

This occurs due to failure of rotation of pancreas surrounding second part of duodenum. Common with Down syndrome. Presents with visible peristalsis, bile stained vomiting if the obstruction is below ampulla of Vater. Treated by bypass (duodenojejunostomy or duodenoduodenostomy). Resection of band may lead to pancreatic fistula.

SAQ 10 What are the causes of iatrogenic pancreatic injury?

Iatrogenic pancreatic injury may occur with:
- During splenectomy
- Billroth II operation
- During enucleation of islet cell tumour
- Sphincterotomy

LAQ 11 Classify pancreatitis?

There are two useful classifications

PANCREATITIS

Etiological

- Alcohol
- Postoperative or traumatic
- In mumps, vascular disease, hyperparathyroidism
- Biliary tract disease

According to presentation

- Acute pancreatitis
- Relapsing acute pancreatitis
- Chronic pancreatitis
- Relapsing chronic pancreatitis

LAQ 12 How acute pancreatitis presents?

- Pain abdomen agonising, generally after heavy meal, (illimitable agony)
- Vomiting and retching
- Rigidity and tenderness
- Shock
- Cyanosis
- Slight jaundice
- Ileus
- A palpable tender mass in 3rd week at epigastrium (pseudocyst) is the important clinical features of pancreatitis.

LAQ 13 How to investigate pancreatitis?

Important tests for pancreatitis are:

- Leukocytosis
- Glycosuria
- Plasma fibrinogen raised
- Renal holo
- CT
- USG
- Raised serum amylase (normal 80–150) Somogyi unit
- Bilirubin slightly raised
- Methaemalbumin in blood (poor prognosis)
- Plain X-ray abdomen (sentinel loop/colon cut off sign)
- Gallstone or pancreatic calcification

LAQ 14 What are the parameters taken for Ranson Score or Glassgow Scale system of pancreatitis?

For Ranson Score	Glasgow Score
Age > 55 years Leukocytosis Raised glucose LDH AST BUN Base deficit Fluid sequestration Low PaO_2 and serum calcium	Age > 55 years Leukocytosis Raised glucose Urea LDH AST Low PaO_2, Ca and albumin

LAQ 15 Name the important complications of pancreatitis.

COMPLICATIONS OF PANCREATITIS

General

Cardiac: (Hypotension, arrhythmia)
Pulmonary: (Oedema; ARDS)
Renal failure
Metabolic: (↓ Ca; Mg; albumin)
Haematological: (DIC: ↓ haematocrit)
Neurological: (Confusion)
GIT (Ileus; fluid sequestration)

Local

- Phlegmon
- Oedema
- Effusion
- Ascitis
- Pseudocyst
- Abscess of pancreas
- Necrosis

LAQ 16 How to manage pancreatitis conservatively?

1. Atropine or propantheline
2. Nasogastric suctions
3. IV infusion
4. 10 ml of 10% calcium gluconate daily
5. Antibiotics

Other: Low molecular weight dextran, hydrocortisone

- Dorsolumbar paravertebral block
- Trasylol (aprotinin—antitryptic substance may be given)
- Glucagon to inhibit pancreatic secretion

LAQ 17 What are the different types of pancreatic cysts?

PANCREATIC CYSTS

True 20%

- Cystadenoma
- Mucoviscidosis
- Congenital cyst
- Retention cyst
- Hydatid cyst

Pseudo 80%

- Collection of fluid in lesser sac treated by cystogastrostomy if conservative treatment fails and cyst is infected.

SAQ 18 What is chronic relapsing pancreatitis?

Here there slow and progressive destruction of acini, fibrosis and pancreatic failure. There may be calcification.

SAQ 19 How chronic pancreatitis presents?

More in men, recurrent pain in epigastrium, once a week or three times a year, which increases in frequency, vomiting, weakness, atherosclerosis.

SAQ 20 Mention the important tests for chronic pancreatitis.

Serum amylase raised during attack.

Stool: Bulky pale, frothy, floats in water.

Steatorrhoea test; Lundh test to determine trypsin actively (normally it is 9μ Eq/min/ml, but in pancreatic steatorrhoea it is less than 2μEq/min/ml.

Glucose tolerance: Glycosuria.

Occult blood in stool is absent in pancreatitis, but positive in Ca pancreas. MRI; CT scan; ERCP; percutaneous pancreatography.

LAQ 21 How to treat chronic pancreatitis?

(i) Low fat (ii) No alcohol (iii) Enzyme supplementation

(iv) Obstruction removal by:

- (a) Pancreatoduodenectomy
- (b) Pancreatojejunostomy
- (c) Cholecystojejunostomy (if there is jaundice)

LAQ 22 How to treat pancreatic fistula?

Pancreatic fistula generally occurs in trauma and is treated by:

(i) Treatment of fluid and electrolyte
(ii) Prevention of autodigestion of skin by 1% HCl in ZnO cream
(iii) Drainage of the discharge
(iv) Surgical
  (a) Fistula drains to stomach (b) Roux-en-Y jejunal loop

SAQ 23 What is insulinoma?

It is beta cell tumour of pancreas, presents with whipple triad.

(i) Effect occurs after fasting (ii) Hypoglycaemia (iii) Relieved by glucose

Treated by extirpation of tumour.

SAQ 24 What are the different types of Zollinger-Ellison syndrome (ZES)?

ZES (type I): Antral G cell hyperplasia, hypergastrinaemia, peptic ulcer (treated by partial gastrectomy).
ZES (type II): Peptic ulcer, hypergastrinaemia, hyperacidity, diarrhoea, steatorrhoea treated by (total gastrectomy with removal of tumour).

LAQ 25 Classify primary pancreatic neoplasia.

PANCREATIC NEOPLASIA

Benign

Epithelial origin Papilloma
Adenoma
Cystadenoma
Serous, mucinous; carcinoid
Oncocytoma

Connective tissue (Fibroma, leiomyoma, neurilemmoma, lymphangioma, haemangioma)

Mixed epithelial and connective (fibroadenoma)

Uncertain histology

Malignant

Epithelial
- Duct cell Ca
- Adenosquamous
- Mucinous, oat cell
- Ciliated cell Ca
- Acinar cell Ca, etc.

Connective tissue
- Fibrosarcoma
- Leiomyosarcoma
- Malignant fibrous histiocytoma

Uncertain
(Pancreatoblastoma, simple or mixed)

SAQ 26 What is the common site of Ca pancreas?

Common in head 70%; in body and tail 30%.

LAQ 27 How a Ca pancreas presents?

Painless progressive jaundice:

- Pain
- Gallbladder palpable (Courvoisier law)
- Anorexia
- Diarrhoea (lead paint)
- Weight loss
- Liver enlargement
- Cholecystitis features

Pain without jaundice when lying, not related to food:

- Weakness, anorexia
- Weight loss
- Diarrhoea.

SAQ 28 How to investigate Ca pancreas?

(i) C loop of barium-filled duodenum is widened (Pad sign) or reverse 3 sign.
(ii) Pancreatic secretion test for Papanicolaou staining
(iii) ERCP
(iv) USG
(v) CT scan

SAQ 29 How will you manage Ca pancreas?

By operative treatment (pancreaticoduodenectomy) preoperative and postoperative vitamin K or palliative operations like cholecystojejunostomy or stenting (if jaundice).

22 Oesophagus

SAQ 1 Describe in brief the anatomy of oesophagus.

Oesophagus is 25 cm long fibromuscular organ extending from cricopharyngeal sphincter to cardiac end of the stomach, occupying posterior mediastinum and below diaphragm. It has three constrictions one at cricopharyngeal constriction, one at the level of arch of arota and one at the level of the diaphragm, lined by squamous epithelium and lower portion by gastric type of mucosa.

SAQ 2 What is dysphagia?

It is difficulty (not the pain) in swallowing.

LAQ 3 How will you investigate dysphagia?

- History
- Clinical types: (with or without pain; dysphagia for solid or liquid food; with regurgitation or not)
- Loss of weight, cachexia, anaemia
- Radiography; Ba swallow
- Oesophagoscopy (rigid; video-oesophagoscopy)
- CT; endoscopic USG
- Motility studies
- 24 hours pH measurement.

SAQ 4 What are the methods to treating dysphagia?

- Dilatation of stricture (eder-dilator; celestin dilator); or ballon dilator.
- Laser therapy to cure a channel for palliation of dysphagia.

SAQ 5 Name some congenital abnormalities of oesophagus.

- Atresia of oesophagus with or without tracheo-oesophageal fistula.
- Stenosis of oesophagus.
- Dysphagia lusoria: Vascular anomaly compressing oesophagus (due to abnormal development of aortic arch or by aberrant right subclavian artery).

SAQ 6 What is Pulsion diverticulum?

This rare variety of diverticulum occurs where blood vessels enter oesophagus generally associated with neuromuscular inco-ordination, presents with dysphagia.

SAQ 7 What is dysphagia lusoria?

Abnormal development of aortic arch producing oesophageal compression by an abnormal artery.

SAQ 8 What is the cause of oesophageal varices?

Portal hypertension.

SAQ 9 What is odynophagia?

It is pain on swallowing.

LAQ 10 What are the causes of oesophagitis?

Causes of oesophagitis

Acute

- Burn
- Infective
- Ryle's tube trauma
- Peptic ulcer

Chronic

- Reflux
- Operation (Roux-en-Y loop) or oesophago-duodenostomy, etc.

SAQ 11 How a reflux oesephagitis presents and diagnosed?

- Pain
- Occult blood in stool
- Heart burn
- Secondary anaemia.
- Dysphagia
- Diagnosed by X-ray and oesophagoscopy

LAQ 12 What are the different types of hiatus hernia?

1. Sliding hernia (portion of stomach and adjacent portion passes into posterior mediastinum)
2. Para-oesophageal or rolling (greater curvature or whole stomach passes to mediastinum)
3. Mixed hiatus hernia

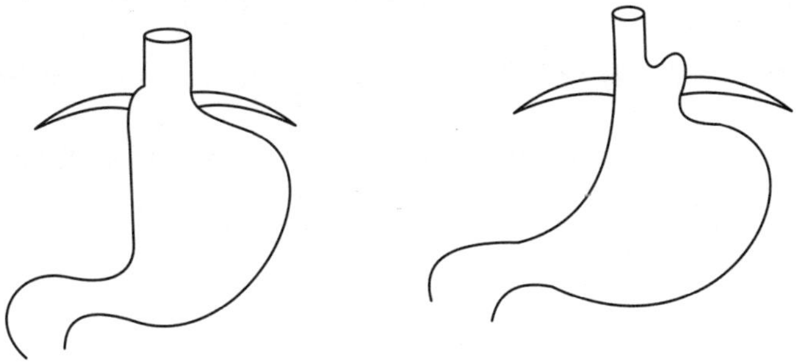

Sliding Paraesophageal

SAQ. 13 What are the indications of surgery in hiatus hernia?

1. Severe symptoms interfering occupation and not controlled by medicine
2. Complications (stenosis, oesophagitis; haemorrhages)
3. Associated lesions like gallstone, ovarian cyst, pyloric ulcer

SAQ 14 What is Boerhaave syndrome?

This is barotrauma of oesophagus where there is perforation of oesophagus when a person vomits against closed glottis.

SAQ 15 What are the causes of perforation of oesophagus?

(i) Barotrauma
(ii) Pathological (Barrett's ulcer)
(iii) Penetrating injury
(iv) Foreign bodies
(v) Oesophagoscopy or instrumentation.

SAQ 16 What is Plummer-Vinson syndrome?

It is characterized by:

Middle-aged women presents with dysphagia, tongue without papillae, pale, inflamed

Lips and corner of mouth are cracked; finger koilonychias, spleen enlarged; hypochromic anemia; bone marrow without iron stores, achlorhydria

LAQ 17 What is cardiospasm or achalasia of oesophagus?

This disease of oesophagus of unknown etiology where oesophageal paristalsis is disorganized and failure of relaxation of cardia.

Different etiologies are: Stress or emotion upset, (vitamin B_1 deficiencies), Chaga's disease (Trypanosomiasis).

Treated by disruption of constriction fibres of cardia, Heller' operation (from without); Plummer's hydrostatic bag (from within).

SAQ 18 What is GORD?

Incompetence of lower oesophageal sphincter producer gastro-oesophageal reflux disease. Reflux oesophagits is a complication of it.

SAQ 19 How a GORD patient presents?

- Retrosternal heart burn particularly after fatty food and lying flat.
- Reflux of food
- Odynophagia with alcohol
- Dysphagia if there is stricture formation.

SAQ 20 What are the different diagnostic tests for GORD?

- Endoscopy
- Manometry
- 24 hours oesophageal pH recording (gold standard for diagnosis)
- Ba swallow and meal studies.

SAQ 21 How to treat GORD?

GORD treatment

Medical

- Sod – aliginate
- Prokinetics (cisapride)
- H_2-blockers
- PPI

Surgery

- Fundoplication (total or partial) (by operation and endoscope)

SAQ 22 What complications may arise out of GORD?

- Shortening of oesophagus
- Barett's oesophagus (metaplastic changes)
- Stricture

LAQ 23 Name the different neoplasms of oesophagus.

Types of oesophageal neoplasm

Benign

- Leiomyoma
- Polyp

Malignant

- Sarcoma (rare)
- Leiomyosarcoma
- Ca oesophagus (Squamous cell; adenocarcinoma)
- Malignant melanoma

SAQ 24 How a Ca oesophagus patient presents?

- Dysphagia
- Weight loss
- Non-specific dyspepsia

SAQ 25 What are the different modes of treatment for Ca oesophagus?

- Radical oesophagectomy
- Chemotherapy
- Radiotherapy
- Laser
- Stenting

SAQ 26 What is nutcracker oesophagus?

Here peristaltic pressure of oesophagus is greater than 180 mm Hg causing chest pain.

SAQ 27 What is Schatzki ring?

This is a circular ring in distal oesophagus, usually at squamocolumnar junction.

SAQ 28 How to treat Monilial oesophagitis?

Monilial oesophagitis is common in patient taking steroids due to *Candida albicans*.

It is treated with nystatin lozenge or other antifungal drugs.

23 Stomach and Duodenum

SAQ. 1 Name the arteries supplying stomach?

(i) Left gastric artery
(ii) Right gastric artery
(iii) Gastroduodenal artery
(iv) Right gastroepiploic artery
(v) Left gastroepiploic artery
(vi) Short gastric or vasa brevia

SAQ 2 By which structure, pyloric canal is distinguished from 1st part of duodenum in living?

By veins of Mayo.

SAQ 3 What are the different types of histological cells found in stomach?

1. Gastric epithelial cells
2. Parietal cells (secretes HCl)
3. Chief cells secret pepsinogen
4. G cells secreting gastrin.

SAQ 4 What are the different phases of gastric acid secretion?

1. **Cephalic phase** by vagal action
2. **Gastric phase** mediated by gastrin
3. **Intestinal phase** by intestinal factors

SAQ 5 Write short note on gastric mucus.

The mucosa of stomach is covered by mucus a viscid secretion underneath which lies a layer of bicarbonate, which forms mechanical barrier to protect mucosa from *H. pylori*; mechanical damage and from irritation from salicylates, alcohol, etc.

SAQ 6 What happens to motor activity in case of fasting?

During fasting, a few minutes of active motor activity is followed absent of motor activities for hours.

SAQ 7 What are the different tests for gastric secretions?

1. Night fasting secretion
2. Maximal acid output by pentagastrin
3. Insulin induced hypoglycaemia causing acid secretion (Hollander's test) 2 IU of soluble insulin (10 kg given IV)
4. RIA technique to asses circulating gastrin

SAQ 8 What are the different peptide hormones and neurotransmitters responsible for gastric secretions?

(a) Neurocrine: Acetylcholine
(b) Endocrine: Gastrin
(c) Paracrine: Histamine

LAQ 9 Name the different investigations done for stomach and duodenum ailment.

- Endoscopy
- Contrast radiology with Ba
- CT scan
- Laparoscopy
- Angiography
- Endoscopic ultrasound
- USG in patient of neoplasia
- MRI
- Gastric emptying studies with radio-isotope lebelled food and meals
- Gastric secretions

SAQ 10 What is hypertrophic pyloric stenosis?

In this condition, there is failure of pylorus to relax causing obstructions. In some cases, there is familial association.

SAQ 11 How a hypertrophic stenosis patient presents?

- Ist male born is commonly affected
- Presents between 3–7 weeks generally on 4th week with forcible projectile vomiting without bile followed by hunger
- Weight loss
- Emaciation and dehydration
- Paristalsis in upper abdomen.

SAQ 12 How to diagnose hypertrophic pyloric stenosis?

- History
- Clinical features
- USG

SAQ 13 How to treat hypertrophic pyloric stenosis?

- Correct metabolic deficit and then
- Surgery (Ramstedt's operation).

SAQ 14 What is congenital duodenal atresia?

In this congential condition, there is stenosis across duodenum at the fusion of fore- and mid-gut. Infant vomits from birth which is bile stained and looses weight. May be diagnosed antenatally by USG (double bubble appearance of stomach). Treated by duodenojejunostomy or duodenoduodenostomy.

SAQ 15 What is peptic ulcer?

It is an ulcer in those parts of GI tract where acid peptic digestion takes place, viz. lesser curvature of stomach; lower oesophagus, 1st part of duodenum; anastomosing site of stomach and duodenum; Mickel's diverticulum.

SAQ 16 How does *H. pylori* produce peptic ulcer?

These bacteria hydrolyse urea, producing strong alkali amonia, which acts on G cells to produce gastrin and hypersecretion of gastric juice. Some strains of *H.pylori* produce cytotoxin Cag A and Vac A which are responsible for chronic gastritis, peptic ulcer and cancer.

LAQ 17 What do you mean by type A and type B gastritis?

The following are the differences between type A and type B gastritis:

Type A gastritis	Type B gastritis
Autoimmune inflammatory condition with circulating antibodies to parietal cells causing atrophy of parietal cells, hypoclorhydria and malabsorption of vitamin B_{12}	It is generally associated with *H.pylori* infection.

LAQ 18 Define the following types of gastritis.

- **Reflux gastritis:** Gastritis due to enterogastric reflux.
- **Erosive gastritis:** Caused by noxious agents disturbing gastric mucosal barrier.
- **Stress gastritis:** Occurs due to stress injury as becuase of less blood supply.
- **Menetrier's disease:** In this premalignant condition, there is hypertrophy of gastric mucosal folds with mucus production and hypochlorhydria. The etiology may be overexpression of transforming growth factor alpha (TGF α). Treated by gastrectomy.
- **Lymphocytic gastritis:** Here gastric mucosa is infiltrated with T cells probably due to *H. pylori* infection.
- **Eosinophilia gastritis:** Gastritis due to allergy, treated by cromoglycate.
- **AIDS gastritis:** Secondary to infection of cryptospiridiosis.
- **Phlegmonous gastritis:** Here rare bacterial infection of stomach occurs due to intercurrent illness.

SAQ 19 Which ulcer is more prone to get malignancy, gastric or duodenal?

Malignancy is common with gastric ulcer.

SAQ 20 Mention the clinical features of peptic ulcer.

- Epigastric intermittent gnawing pain, may radiate to back, food relieves it. It is periodic
- Vomiting if stenosis
- Weight gain or loss
- Haematemesis or melaena

SAQ 21 Mention the important investigations of peptic ulcer.

Nowadays gastroduodenoscopy with antral biopsy to determine *H. pylori* infection.

SAQ 22 How will you treat peptic ulcer?

- Lifestyle modification (stop smoking)
- H_2 receptor blocker and/or PPI
- Eradication of *H. pylori* with amoxycillin/azithromycin/tinidazole/metronidazole/tetracycline.

LAQ 23 Name the different operations of peptic ulcer.

AIMS of operation

Gastric ulcer

- Excision of ulcer bearing area
- Improve stomach emptying
- Prevent complications and remove malignancy

Duodenal ulcer

- Reduce acid contact and reduce acid secretion
- Prevent complications

Different operations for duodenal ulcers are:

- Bilroth II operation
- Gastrojejunostomy
- Truncal vagotomy with drainage (pyloroplasty; gastrojejunostomy)
- Highly selective vagotomy
- Turncal vagotomy with antrectomy (source of gastrin is removed)

Operations for gastric ulcers:

- Bilroth type I gastrectomy
- Bilroth type II gastrectomy
- Vagotomy, pyloroplasty and ulcer excision.

LAQ 24 What complications may arise out of chronic peptic ulcer?

Complication of peptic ulcer

Acute

- Perforation
- Haematemesis and melaena

Subacute

- Residual obscess

Chronic

- Stenosis (pyloric teapot, hourglass,
- Penetration
- Cancer

SAQ 25 What is Mallory-Weiss syndrome?

Male over 50 years presents with prolonged vomiting, starts vomiting blood, generally after taking alcohol due to longitudinal tear below gastro-oesophageal junction.

LAQ 26 Name the important complications after gastric operations.

The important complications arise after gastric operations are as follows:

General complications

- Anaesthetic (pulmonary; cardiac thrombotic)

Specific complications

Early

- Haemorrhage
- Paralytic ileus
- Obstruction of stomach
- Duodenal fistula
- Pancreatitis

Late

- Recurrence
- Fistula (gastro-jejunocolic)
- Post-gastrotomy syndrome
- Tuberculosis
- Anemia
- Gallstone
- Cancer
- Intestinal obstruction

LAQ 27 Name the different post-gastrectomy syndrome.

Postcibal syndrome

- Early
  - Dumping
- Late
  - Hypoglycaemia
- Bilious vomiting

Nutritional syndrome

- Steatorrhoea
- Weight loss
- Diarrhoea
- Iron deficiency anaemia
- Megaloblastic anaemia
- Malabsorption

LAQ 28 What do you mean by postcibal syndrome?

These syndromes occur after gastrotomy. It may be: (i) early, (ii) late postcibal syndrome.

Early postcibal syndrome	Late postcibal syndrome
Syndrome consisting of abdominal and vasomotor symptoms due to rapid emptying of stomach. Fall in blood volume. **Symptoms are:** Epigastric fullness, tachycardic sweating, feeling warm, colic and diarrhoea occurs after food. Precipitated by bulk of food and relieved by lying down.	This serious complication occurs due to hypoglycaemia, due to increased insulin hypersensibility, due to hyperglycaemia. **Presenting symptoms are:** Tremer, nausea, epigastric emptiness, fainting occurs two hours after food. Aggravated by exercise and relieved by food or glucose.

SAQ 29 How will you treat post-vagotomy diarrhoea?

This condition is difficult to treat. Following drugs are given:

- Codeine phosphate
- Course of phthalylsulphathiazole
- Neomycin
- Revisional surgery

SAQ 30 What is Dieulafoy's disease?

This is gastric arterial venous malformation presents with bleeding.

SAQ 31 What are the macroscopical varieties of gastric carcinoma?

The Ca stomach is captain of men of death, may present as following types macroscopically.

- **Type I** : Cauliflower-like growth with sharp well-defined edge
- **Type II** : Ulcer with irregular indurated edge
- **Type III** : Colloid carcinoma
- **Type I** : Scirrhous type
- **Type V** : Carcinoma secondary to chronic gastric ulcer.

SAQ 32 What are the different modes of spread of Ca stomach?

- Direct spread
- Lymphatic (permeation, emboli)
- Blood-borne (liver, lung, bone)
- Transperitoneal (Krukenberg's tumour)

SAQ 33 What is Krukenberg's tumour and Sister Joseph nodule?

Spread of gastric carcinoma to ovaries is called Krukenberg's tumour and when it spreads to umbilicus it is Sister Joseph nodule.

SAQ 34 What is Zollinger-Ellison syndrome?

These are gastrin producing tumour generally in duodenal loops or pancreatic head.

SAQ 35 Name the different operations performed for obesity.

(i) Vertical banded gastroplasty
(ii) Gastric bypass operation
(iii) Placing an inflatable band around upper stomach distal to oesophagogastric junction by laparo scope in tried.

SAQ 36 What is trichobezoar and phytobezoar?

Trichobezoar are hair balls found in stomach generally in female psychiatric patient, presents with ulcer, bleeding, perforation or obstruction.

Phytobezoar is vegetables in stomach due to gastric stasis.

SAQ 37 What is volvulus of stomach?

Here stomach rotates between two fixed points cardia and pylorus, treated by operations.

24 Peritoneum

SAQ 1 What are the different layers of peritoneum?

(i) **Visceral**: Surrounding the viscera.
(ii) **Parietal**: Lining the cavities.

SAQ 2 What are causes of acute peritonitis?

- **Bacterial infection** (appendicitis)
- **Chemial injury** (bile peritonitis)
- **Ischaemic injury** (strangulation of bowel)
- **Direct trauma** (penetrating wound or operational peritonitis)
- **Allergy** (starch peritonitis)

SAQ 3 How bacteria enters peritoneum?

Bacteria enters peritoneum by:

(i) **Direct infection** (perforation, penetration, operation)
(ii) **Local extension** (inflamed organ or gut wall or via fallopian tube)
(iii) **Blood** (septicaemia)
(iv) **Exogenous contamination** (drain, open surgery)

SAQ 4 Name bacteria involved in peritonitis.

Bacteria from:

GI source (*E. coli; Strepto, Staphylo, Bacteroides, Clostridium, Klebsiella*);

Other sources (*Chlamydia, Gonococcus; β-haemolytic Strepto, Pneumo, Mycobacterium tuberculosis*)

LAQ. 5 How a peritonitis patient presents?

Clinical presentation of peritonitis

Localised peritonitis

- Pain abdomen (may be refd. to shoulder)
- Repeated vomiting
- Tender abdomen with gaurding
- Rise of pulse and tempcrature
- Absent paristalsis

Generalised peritonitis

Early

- Pain worse on movement or breathing
- Vomiting
- Gaurding or tenderness
- Urinary symptoms in pelvic variety
- Paralytic ileus.

Intermediate

- Peritonitis resolve so
- Pain diminishes
- Pulse slow
- Silent, soft abdomen

Late

- Abdomen silent
- Distended
- Cold skin
- Circulatory failure
- Unconsci-ousness

LAQ 6 What is acute abdomen? Mention the important causes of acute abdomen.

Acute abdomen is any condition giving rise to acute abdominal pain may require operation

Causes of acute abdomen

Intraabdominal

- Appendicitis
- Pancreatitis
- Cholecystitis
- Salpingitis
- Peritonitis
- Diverticulitis
- Peptic or typhoid perforation
- Intestinal obstruction (stone faecolith, stricture, round worm, paralytic ileus)
- Hirschsprung's disease
- Mesenteric thrombosis
- Ectopic gestation rupture
- Rupture spleen
- Twisted ovarian or spleen pedicle
- Colics (biliary, appendix, renal, intestinal)

Extraabdominal

Thoracic

- Pneumonia
- Diaphragmatic pleurisy
- Pneumothorax
- Angina

Retroperitoneal

- Pyelitis
- Dietl's crisis
- Aneurysm of aorta
- Retroperitoneal lymphangitis

SAQ 7 Mention the important investigations of peritonitis.

- Leukocytosis
- Raised serum amylase
- Gas under diaphragm if hollow viscus perforation in erect posture
- USG
- Perineal fluid aspiration

LAQ 8 How will you treat peritonitis?

Treatment of peritonitis

General care of patient

- Correction of fluid and electrolyte balance
- Nasogastric secretion
- Vital system support
- Analgesia (morphine)
- Antibiotics

Specific treatment

- Treat the cause like peptic ulcer, appendicitis

Peritoneal lavage

- Explore peritoneal cavity with sucker
- Mop up dry to remove seropurulent exudate

LAQ 9 What may complications arise out of peritonitis?

(i) Abdominal complications:

- Adhesion
- Portal pyemia
- Paralytic ileus
- Liver abscess
- Recurrent abscess

(ii) Systemic complications:

- Bacteremic shock
- Renal failure
- Multisystem failure
- Pneumonia
- Bone marrow suppression
- Respiratory failure

SAQ 10 What are the causes of pelvic abscess?

- Appendicular disease
- Fallopian tube disease or following large bowel or rectal surgery

SAQ 11 What are the causes of subphrenic abscess?

Subphrenic abscess causes

Left subphrenic	Right subphrenic	Right subhepatic	Periphrenic abscess
Boundary: Above diaphragm behind left triangular ligament and left lobe. Causes: Operation of stomach, Tail of pancreas, spleen (splenic flexure)	Space between right lobe of liver and diaphragm to the left by falciforrm ligament posterioly by anterior layer of right triangular ligament Causes: Perforated duodenal ulcer; appendicitis.	Space between Right lobe of liver and to left foramen of Winslow and below by duodenum. Causes: Appendicitis, cholecystitis, duodenal ulcer perforation, upper abdominal surgery	Boundary: Bare area. Causes: Amoebic liver abscess.

Aphorism: Pus somewhere, pus to where, it is under diaphragm.

LAQ 12 How subphrenic abscess presents? How will you investigate it?

Clinical features of subphrenic abscess

Symptoms

- History of infection in abdomen
- Sweating
- Anorexia
- Epigastric fullness and pain
- Hiccough

Signs

- Temperature
- Tenderness
- Rigidity
- Palpable swelling
- Collapse lungs
- Basal effusion

Investigations

(i) Leukocytosis,
(ii) Radiology (presence of gas or pleural effusion, tented diaphragm)
(iii) USG; CT
(iv) Radiolabelled white cell scanning.

SAQ 13 What are the causes of bile peritonitis?

- Perforated cholecystitis
- Post-cholecystectomy
- T-tube drain dislodgement
- Following other operations involving gallbladder

SAQ 14 What are the sources of tuberculosis infection in peritoneum?

- Tuberculosis mesenteric lymph node
- Ileocaecal tuberculosis
- Salpingitis (Tb)
- Blood-borne (miliary)

SAQ 15 What are the different types of tuberculosis peritonitis?

- Ascitic
- Encysted
- Fibrous
- Purulent

LAQ 16 What are the causes of ascites?

Ascites causes

Transudate (< 25 g protein/L)

- Low plasma protein (malnutrition; nephrotic syndrome, protein losing malnutrition)
- CCF
- Cirrhosis and portal venous thrombosis

Exudate (> 25 gm/L)

- Tuberculosis of peritoneum
- Malignancy of peritoneum
- Budd-Chiari syndrome
- Pancreatic
- Chylous
- Meigs' syndrome

SAQ 17 What are the causes of chylous ascites?

Ascitic fluid is milky due to excess chylomicrons:

- Malignant (lymphoma)
- Cirrhosis
- Filariasis
- Nephrotic syndrome
- Trauma of abdomen
- Sacroidosis
- Constrictive pericarditis
- Congenital lymphatic defect

SAQ 18 What is peritoneal mice?

These are loose bodies rarely causing symptoms, viz. appendix epiploica. These are of pea size contain saponified fat surrounded by fibrins.

SAQ 19 Name some neoplasms of peritoneum.

Some neoplasms of peritoneum are following:

- Carcinoma peritonei
- Psudomyxoma peritonei (in cystic tumour of ovary and rupture of mucocele of the appendix)
- Desmoid (familial adenomatous polyposis)
- Mesothelioma

SAQ 20 Mention some indications of laparoscopic surgery.

It is done for **diagnostic** (ascites, liver metastasis, staging neoplasm, acute abdomen) **Therapeutic** for abdominal operations.

SAQ 21 What is seat belt syndrome?

If a person sitting in a car with seat belt worn, and car undergone sudden deceleration may tear mesentery called seat belt syndrome.

LAQ 22 What are the different types of mesenteric cyst?

Mesenteric cyst

Chylolymphatic	Enterogenous	Urogenital	Miscellaneous
• Congenital misplaced lymphatic tissue	• Derives from diverticulum of mesenteric border of intestine or from duplicated intestine	• Wolffian or mullerian	• Dermoid • Serosanguinous • Hydatid

SAQ 23 How a mesenteric cyst presents?

A painless abdominal swelling near umbilicus moving right angles to attachments of mesentery.

or

Recurrent abdominal pain with or without vomiting or acute abdomen due to torsion, rupture haemorrhage.

SAQ 24 Name some neoplasms of mesentery.

It may be: (i) **Benign** (lipoma, fibroma, fibromyxoma)

(ii) **Malignant** (lymphoma or secondary carcinoma reticulosarcoma)

25 Intestine (Small and Large)

SAQ 1 What is Hirschsprung's disease?

Here there is congenital absence of ganglion in myoenteric plexus of distal hind gut (short or long segment).

SAQ 2 How Hirschsprung's disease presents and diagnosed and treated?

- Passage of meconium beyond 24 hours.
- Abdominal distension
- Bilious vomiting
- Enterocolitis
- Chronic constipation in first few weeks.

Diagnosis

(a) Rectal biopsy showing aganglionosis and hypertropic nerve fibres in the plexus.
(b) Rectal manometry
(c) Radiology

Treatment

For short segment (myomectomy)

For long segment, the operations are:

(a) Duhamel operation
(b) Swenson's operation
(c) Coloanal anastomosis
(d) Restrorative proctocolectomy

SAQ 3 What is idiopathic slow transit constipation?

This condition is generally occurs in women, cannot empty rectum normally. Either present since childhood or after abdominal or pelvic surgery.

SAQ 4 What is angiodysplasia of gut?

This is a vascular malformation associated with aging commonly in ascending colon and caecum. May be with cutaneous or oral vascular malformation of hereditary telangiectasia. These are dilated distorted thin walled vessels with little muscle in vessel walls. Diagnosed by colonoscopy and radioactive technetium 99m lebelled RBC or transillumination through caecum.

SAQ 5 What effect is produced by blind loop syndrome?

In blind loop syndrome, stasis causes abnormal gut flora leading to defective absorption. Antibiotics cause temporary relief. If it occurs in upper intestine, defect in fat absorption occurs. Lower intestinal defect manifests as vitamin B_{12} deficiency and anemia.

SAQ 6 What are the different types of diverticular diseases?

It may be ***congenital*** (all coats of bowel present in diverticulum), ***acquired*** (lack of muscular coat).

SAQ 7 What are the types of duodenal diverticulum?

Primary (on older patient) and ***secondary*** (in duodenal cap of duodenal ulcer patient)

LAQ 8 What is Meckel's diverticulum?

It is congenital diverticulum found in 2% of patients, situated 2 feet from ileocaecal junction, 2 inches in length, containing functional gastric mucosa.

It may cause:

- Haemorrhage
- Diverticulitis
- Intestinal obstruction.
- Intussusception
- Peptic ulcer

It is frequently suspected, often sought, but rarely found. It may be found in inguinal and femoral hernia (Littre's hernia).

SAQ 9 What is diverticula?

It is acquired herniation of colonic mucosa protruding circular muscle at the point where blood vessels penetrates the gut wall. It is probably due to muscular incoordination, spasm which increases guts intraluminal pressure.

LAQ 10 What is diverticulitis? How it presents and diagnosed? What are its complications?

Inflammation of one or more diverticula may be asymptomatic or presents within lower abdominal pain, pain left iliac fossa, with distension, flatulence and heaviness of lower abdomen. Constipation or loose motion. Palpable tender thickend sigmoid colon may be there. There may urinary symptoms with vesico-colic fistula.

Diagnosed by exclusion (colonoscopy; CT): Ba radiology

Complications

- Diverticulitis
- Haemorrhage
- Pericolitis and abscess
- Fistula
- Peritonitis

Management: High residue diet: Acute diverticulitis by rest and IV antibiotics (ceforoxime and metronidazole). Operations are required if there is recurrence or complications.

LAQ 11 How Ca colon differs from diverticulitis?

Ca colon	Diverticulitis
Short history	Long history
Less common	More common
Painless mass	Painful tender mass
Small persisting bleeding	Profuse bleeding
Localised change in X-ray	Diffuse change in X-ray
No inflammatory change if there is no ulcer in sigmoidoscopy	Sigmoidoscopy shows inflammatory change

LAQ 12 What is the probable hypothesis of ulcerative colitis?

Ulcerative colitis is a disease of unknown etiology, starts in rectum and spread proximally. Probable hypotheses are:

- Mucosal immunological reaction
- Weakened mucosal barrier
- Defective mucosal metabolism of butarate
- Smoking or chewing nicotine causes remission.

SAQ 13 How an ulcerative colitis presents?

- Pain (with relapse or remission)
- Bloody or watery diarrhoea
- Mucosal discharge either blood-stained or purulent

SAQ 14 How the disease severity of ulcerative colitis is determined clinically?

- More than 4 motions/day
- Fever
- Tachycardia
- Hypoaluminaemia

SAQ 15 What are the complications of ulcerative colitis?

- Fulminating colitis
- Perforation
- Rectal bleeding
- Skin lesions (erythema nodosum, aphthous ulcer, pyoderma gangrenosum)
- Eye (iritis)
- Liver (sclerosing cholangitis)
- Cancer

LAQ 16 How to treat ulcerative colitis?

Treatment of ulcerative colitis

Medical

Mild: Prednisolone 20–40 mg/day sulfasalazine 1 gm TDS
Severe: Nothing per month and rectal prednisolone, azathioprine or cyclosporin

Surgery

- Protocolectomy and ileostomy
- Rectal and anal dissection
- Restorative protocolectomy with ileo anal pouch
- Colectomy and iliorectal anastomosis
- Ileostomy with continent intraabdominal pouch.

LAQ 17 What is regional enteritis (Crohn's disease)?

This chronic inflammatory disease may affect any part of GIT from lip to anus but common in ileum. Rejection specimen shows:

- Fibrosis of the lumen
- Snake-like deep mucosal ulceration
- Adhesion
- Fistula with adjacent structures.
- Dilatation proximal to stricture
- Oedema of mucosa like cobblestone appearance
- Mesenteric abscess and lymph node enlargement
- Microscopically, all the layers of intestinal walls are involved and there is non-caseating giant cell granuloma.

SAQ 18 Name the important investigations of Crohn's disease.

Barium enema (string sign)

- Sonogram
- CT scan MRI for assessing perianal diseases.
- Sigmoidoscope or colonoscopy

LAQ 19 How a Crohn's disease presents?

Presentation of Crohn's disease

Acute

- Diarrhoea
- Like appendicitis
- Toxic megacolon

Chronic

- Pain right iliac fossa
- Tender mass
- Fistula
- Growth retardation
- Food fear in children

LAQ 20 How to treat Crohn's disease?

Medical

- Prednisolone
- 5-ASA compounds
- Antibiotics for abscess
- Nutritional support

Surgery

Indications:
- Intestinal obstruction
- Perforation or bleeding
- Fistula
- Failure of medical treatment
- Perianal disease
- Malignancy

Operations are:
- Ileocaecal resection
- Segmental resection
- Colectomy and ileorectal anastomosis
- Strictureplasty
- Temporary loop jejunostomy
- Proctocolectomy
- Drainage of anal abscess.

LAQ 21 How ulcerative colitis differs from Crohn's disease?

Following are the differences between ulcerative colitis and Crohn's disease:

Ulcerative colitis (UC)	Crohn's disease (CD)
1. Affects colon	Any GI part is affected
2. Mucosal disease	effects full thickness
3. Confluent lesion	Skip lesions
4. Stricture and fistula less common	More common
5. No granuloma found	Granuloma found
6. Not so	Affects terminal ileum
7. No recurrence after resection	Recurrence occurs after resection

SAQ 22 What are the surgical complications of typhoid and paratyphoid?

(i) Cholecystitis
(ii) Phlebitis
(iii) Cystitis, pyelitis, epididymo-orchitis
(iv) Arthritis
(v) Osteomyelitis
(vi) Paralytic ileus
(vii) Intestinal haemorrhage
(viii) Perforation

LAQ 23 What are the different types of tuberculosis of intestine? How they present?

Types

Ulcerative type	Hyperplastic type
Presents with • Diarrhoea • Weight loss	• Abdominal pain • Intermittent diarrhoea • Mass in iliac fossa
Diagnosis: Ba meal	Ba meal

Treatment: ATD and surgery, if obstruction.

SAQ 24 How to treat actinomycosis of ileocaecal region?

With high dose of penicillin and or cotrimoxazole for prolong period.

SAQ 25 What is Peutz-Jeghers syndrome?

Familial polyposis: causing haemorrhage, intussusception and melanosis of mucous membrane and lips.

SAQ 26 Name some benign tumours of small intestine.

- Adenoma
- Submucous lipoma
- Stromal cell tumours

SAQ 27 Name some malignant disease of small intestine.

- Lymphoma
- Carcinoma
- Carcinoid tumour

LAQ 28 What are the different types of polyp of large intestine?

Polyp is elevated tumour. It may of following varieties in large intestine.

- **Infammatory**
- **Metaplastic**
- **Hamartoma**
  - Peutz-Jeghers
  - Juvenile polyp
- **Neoplastic**
  - Adenoma
  - Adenocarcinoma
  - Carcinoid tumours

SAQ 29 What are the different macroscopic types of Ca colon?

It may be:

- Annular
- Ulcerative
- Tubular
- Cauliflower types

SAQ 30 Which portion of large gut is more prone to cancer?

Rectum> Sigmoid colon > Caecum

SAQ 31 How Ca colon spreads?

By
- Local
- Lymphatic
- Blood vessels

SAQ 32 How colon cancer is classified?

By Duke's TNM classification. But basic form is:

(a) Confined to bowel wall
(b) Involving peritoneum
(c) Lymph node involvement

Ro = No residual tumour and R_1 = Residual tumour presents

SAQ 33 What are the different methods of diagnosis of Ca colon?

- Sigmoidoscopy
- Double contrast barium meal
- Colonoscopy
- USG

LAQ 34 What operations are done for Ca colon?

For Ca caecum: Peritoneum lateral to ascending colon is incised around hepatic flexure.

Involving transverse colon: Two flexures with transverse mesocolon and greater omentum are incised.

Involving splenic flexure: Right colon and descending colon are cut. Ileorectal anastomosis is done.

Ca pelvic colon: Inferior mesenteric artery below left colonic branch together with paracolic lymph node is resected.

SAQ 35 How the following Ca colon manifest clinically?

Ca left sided colon: Pain, altered bowel habit, lump, distension.
Ca sigmoid colon: Pain, tenesmus, bladder symptoms.
Ca caecum: Anaemia, right iliac fossa mass, intussusception.

SAQ 36 What is pneumatosis cystoides intestinalis?

These are gas filled, translucent cyst. 1 × 2 cm found in subserosa and submucosa of small intestine or colon. May be treated by 70% oxygen continuously for 5 days if producing symptoms and with antibiotics.

SAQ 37 What is colostomy?

It is an artificial opening made on large gut for passing faeces and flatus and collected by external appliances.

It may be:

- Temporary
- Double barreled
- Permanent

SAQ 38 What are the different causes of failure of healing of faecal fistula?

- Presence of active disease
- Associated complex abscess
- Epithelial continuity between gut and skin.

26 Intestinal Obstruction

LAQ 1 What are the types of intestinal obstructions?

Intestinal obstruction

- **Dynamic**: Against mechanical obstruction
- **Adynamic**: No mechanical elements, viz. paralytic ileus, vascular occlusion

SAQ 2 What are the types of dynamic obstruction?

It may occur in small bowel (high or low) or large bowel obstruction.

LAQ 3 Mention the important causes of intestinal obstruction?

Intestinal obstruction causes

- **Dynamic**
  - **Luminal**
    - Gallstone
    - Impaction
    - Foreign bodies
  - **Mural**
    - Stricture
    - Malignancy
  - **Extramural**
    - Bands
    - Hernia
    - Volvulus
    - Intussusception
- **Adynamic**
  - Paralytic ileus
  - Pseudo-obstruction
  - Mesenteric vascular occlusion

SAQ 4 What is closed loop obstruction?

Here bowel is obstructed at proximal and distal points.

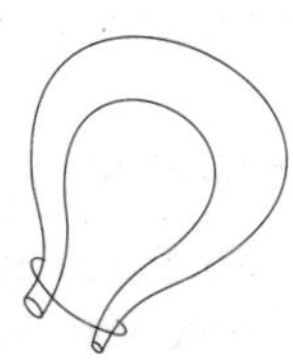

SAQ 5 What is strangulation of intestine?

In this variety of intestinal obstruction, the viability of bowel is threatened by compromised blood supply. Causes are:

- Hernia
- Volulus
- Intussusception
- Closed loop obstruction
- Mesenteric infarction.

SAQ 6 How intestinal obstruction presents?

- Pain
- Distension
- Vomiting
- Obstipation
- Dehydration
- Fever
- Hypokalaemia
- Pyrexia
- Tender abdomen.

SAQ 7 Name the conditions where constipation may not be present in intestinal obstruction.

- Ritcher's hernia
- Gallstone obstruction
- Mesenteric vascular occlusions
- Pelvic abscess
- Partial obstruction (faecal impaction)

SAQ 8 What are the clinical features of strangulation?

Strangulation is surgical emergency. It is diagnosed clinically by:

(i) Features of shock
(ii) Pain
(iii) Tenderness and rigidity

SAQ 9 What are the radiological features of intestinal obstruction?

Errect and straight abdomen X-ray shows:

- Jejunum is seen by its conniventes
- Multiple fluid levels are seen later
- Obstructed intestine is straight segment lie transversly
- Haustral folds are seen in large intestine.
- Jejunum, ileum and caecum are distended with gas.

SAQ 10 What is the principle of treating intestinal obstruction?

Ryle's or Salem tube for nasogastric suction

(i) Fluid and electrolyte replacement (by Hartmann's solution or normal saline)
(ii) Releif of obstruction (note site, nature, cause of obstruction)

SAQ 11 How to differentiate viable and non-viable intestine?

In viable intestine: When hot mop is applied, its colour becomes lighter, mesentery bleeds on pricking, omentum is shiny, intestinal muscle is firm and peristalsis can be seen but in **non-viable** intestine, reverse is the case.

LAQ 12 What are the different causes of adhesion of abdomen? How they can be prevented? How to treat recurrent adhesions?

Cause of adhesions:

- Trauma
- Vascular occlusion
- Infection
- Drugs (paractol)
- Raw areas
- Foreign material (silk, talc, etc.)
- Crohn's disease
- Radiation enteritis

Prevention of peritoneal adhesion: Remove clot and wash peritoneal cavity with normal saline; minimize contact of gauze, cover raw peritoneal surfaces.

Treatment of recurrent adhesion:

(i) Enterolysis
(ii) Noble plication operation
(iii) Charles-Phillips transmesenteric plication
(iv) Bakers tube insertion via Witzel jejunostomy

SAQ 13 Name some varieties of bolus obstruction.

- Worms
- Trichobezoars (hairs)
- Stercolith
- Gallstone
- Phytobezoar (vegetable or fruits)

SAQ 14 Name the potential sites of hernia causing intestinal obstruction.

(i) Hole in mesentery and transverse colon
(ii) Foramen of Winslow
(iii) Defects in broad ligaments
(iv) Diaphragmatic hernia, etc.

SAQ 15 What is intussusception?

Here one segment of the gut invaginates in immediate adjacent portion (proximal into distal) It composed of three parts:

(i) Inter tube (intussusceptum)
(ii) Middle returning tube
(iii) Outer tube (intussuscipiens).

SAQ 16 How intussusception presents in children?

- Screaming and drawing up of legs
- Vomiting
- Red current jelly stool
- Emptiness of right iliac fossa (sign of Dance)
- Apex of intussusception may be felt per rectum
- Abdominal distension
- Barium enema may show claw sign.

SAQ 17 What is volvulus?

It is twisting or axial rotation of a portion of gut about its mesentery.

SAQ 18 What is arrested rotation?

Gut lies outside abdominal cavity up to 10th weeks of gestation and returns to abdomen gradually. This return may be arrested at any stage called arrested rotation.

SAQ 19 What is meconium ileus?

Meconium is normally kept fluid by the action of pancreatic enzymes. In cystic fibrosis, it may produce intestinal obstruction called meconium ileus.

SAQ 20 What is paralytic ileus?

In paralytic ileus, there is failure of transmission of peristaltic wave secondary to neuromuscular failure of Auerbach and Meissner plexus.

Treatment

- Nasogastric suction
- Electrolyte balance
- Adrenergic blockers with cholinergic stimulation (catchpole regimen).

SAQ 21 What are the causes of chronic intestinal obstruction?

Important causes are:

- Faeceal impaction
- Diverticulitis
- Adhesion
- Hirschprung's disease
- Colorectal cancer
- Anastomotic stenosis
- Endometriosis

SAQ 22 What is pseudo-intestinal obstruction?

Obstruction of colon in absence of mechanical or acute intraabdominal disease, viz. diabetes, uraemia, myxoedema, myocardial infarction, burn, retroperitoneal irritation (blood, enzymes in pancreatitis, tumour), drugs (levodopa, phenothiazine), Chaga's disease, scleroderma, etc.

SAQ 23 Why acute mesenteric ischaemia is less common in inferior mesenteric artery?

It is because of better collateral supply.

LAQ 24 What are the causes of superior mesenteric artery ischaemia?

Common causes of superior mesenteric artery embolisation are:

(i) Atrial fibrillation
(ii) Atheromatous plaque
(iii) Myocardial infarct
(iv) Mitral vegetation of endocarditis

Causes of superior mesenteric thrombosis are:

- Portal hypertension and pyaemia
- OCP
- Sickle cell disease

27 Vermiform Appendix

SAQ 1 What is the position of the base of appendix?

This constantly present at the confluence of three taeniae coli of the caecum.

LAQ 2 What are the etiologies of acute appendicitis?

Race: More in Europian.

Diet: Low fibres and increased consumption of refined carbohydrate

Social status: More in upper middle class

Familial susceptibility

Obstruction of appendicular lumen (faecolith, stricture, worms)

Use of purgatives: May perforate appendix

Epidemic form: Streptococcal infection entering via nasopharynx.

SAQ 3 What are the different anatomical positions of appendix?

- Retrocaecal
- Paracaecal
- Pre- and post-ileal
- Pelvic
- Subcaecal

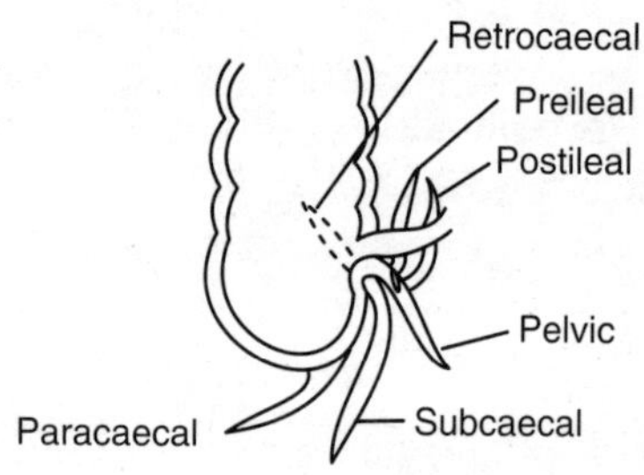

SAQ 4 Name the different congenital anomalies of appendix.

- Agenesis
- Double appendix
- Left sided appendix

SAQ 5 What are the different types of acute appendicitis?

(i) Nonobstructive acute appendicitis
(ii) Obstructive acute appendicitis

LAQ 6 How an appendicitis patient presents?

Acute appendicitis

Non-obstructive

No age is exempted, rare before 2 years and in older age group
Pain abdomen: Umbilicus, epigastrium, generalized or right iliae fossa, pain increases on coughing
Upset of gastric function: Nausea, vomiting foul breath, brown furred tongue
Localised tenderness at McBurney's point, pyrexia, tachycardia, leukocytosis

Obstructive

Vomiting, right iliac fossa tender, other features depend upon site of appendix

SAQ 7 What is Murphy's triad?

The feature of pain, temperature and vomiting is called Murphy's triad.

SAQ 8 What is McBurney's point?

It is point at line joining anterior superior iliac spine and umbilicus at its lateral third with medial two-thirds.

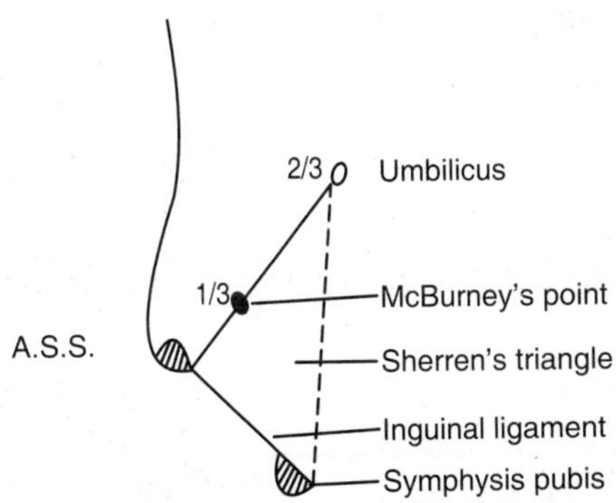

SAQ 9 What is the fate of acute appendicitis?

- Surgical removal
- Peritonitis
- Mucocele
- Resolution
- Appendicular abscess
- Gangrene and perforation
- Fibrosis

SAQ 10 What is Sherren's triangle?

Triangle formed by the point of symphysis pubis, umbilicus and anterior superior iliac spine, sometimes hyperaesthesia may be found over the triangle in appendicitis.

SAQ 11 What is Rovsing's sign?

Pressure on left iliac fossa causing pain at appendix in acute appendicitis.

SAQ 12 What is Cope's psoas test and Cope's obturator test?

Cope's psoas test: Attempt to extend hip causes pain in appendicular area in retrocaecal appendicitis.

Cope's obturator test: Attempt of flex and rotate internally of hip, causes pain in appendicular site in pelvic variety of appendicitis.

LAQ 13 Write down the differential diagnosis of appendix.

Attic: Tonsillitis, pneumonia, pleurisy

Diaphragm to umbilicus: Peptic perforation; acute cholecystitis

Umbilicus to pelvis: Enterocolitis; mesenteric lymphadenitis; Crohn's disease; intestinal obstruction; Meckel's diverticulum; Ca caecum

Pelvis: Salpingitis; ectopic pregnancy; twisted right ovarian cyst; rupture ovarian follicle.

Retroperitoneal: Pyelonephritis; ureteric colic

Other: Herpetic, tabetic, porphyria, pancreatitis, diabetic abdomen

SAQ 14 Mention the important preoperative test for appendicitis.

- Routine TBC and urinalysis
- Urea
- X-ray abdomen
- Pregnancy (female)
- Electrolyte
- USG and CT of abdomen

SAQ 15 How to treat appendicitis?

Immediate appendicectomy for acute appendicitis either by conventional method or by laparoscopy.

SAQ 16 Write down the important differential diagnoses of appendix mass (appendicular phlegmon).

- Appendix abscess
- Crohn's disease
- Twisted ovarian cyst
- Ca caecum
- Parametritis
- Iliac lymphadenitis

SAQ 17 How to treat appendicular abscess?

Immediate drainage and antibiotics. Appendicectomy is performed when abscess dries up otherwise there is chance of fistula formation.

SAQ 18 What is mucocele of appendix?

Here proximal end of the luman of appendix is slowly accluded by fibrous stricture and retains the secretions, which is sterile, causing enlargement of appendix. If it is infected, it becomes empyema of appendix.

SAQ 19 Name some neoplasms of appendix.

- Carcinoid tumour
- Primary adenocarcinoma

SAQ 20 When to stop delayed treatment in appendicular abcess?

- Rising pulse rate
- Abdominal pain spreading
- Copious vomiting
- Size of the abscess increasing

28 Rectum and Anal Canal

SAQ 1 What is the anatomical importance of dentate line?

- It is the fusion site of proctodeum and post-allantoic gut.
- Lined by cubical epithelium above and squamous epithelium below
- Supplied by insensitive autonomic nerves above and sensitive spinal nerves below.
- Drained by portal veins above and systemic veins below.

SAQ 2 Name the different congenital anomalies of rectum and anal canal.

1. **Imperforate anus**
2. **Low abnormalities:** • Covered anus • Ectopic anus • Stenosed anus • Membranous anus
3. **High abnormalities:** • Anorectal agenesis • Rectal atresia • Cloaca (bowel, bladder and genital tracts open by single cavity in women)

SAQ 3 Write short note on sacrococcygeal teratoma.

It is rare tumour, seen in first three months of life. It is the site of primitive knot (totepotent cell) more common in female, arises between sacrum and rectum attached to coccyx at the time of birth, may cause stillbirth. May turn malignant. It should be removed as soon as detected to prevent malignant changes.

LAQ 4 Write short note on pilonidal sinus.

Theory of origin

(i) Congenital
(ii) Post anal dermoid
(iii) Caudal persistant of remnant of neural canal.

Acquired

(i) Occupational more in male
(ii) Occurs in 20–30 years of age with projecting dead hairs
(iii) Hair never seen in the walls
(iv) Recurrence common

Treatment

Conservative: Clean the track, avoid long sitting in cars; antibiotics

Operative: Incise the abscess or operation for marsupialization of sinus; skin grafting

Cause of recurrence

(i) A diverticulum is overlooked
(ii) New hair entering scar
(iii) Trauma

SAQ 5 What is fissure in ano?

It is an elongated ulcer along the long axis of lower anal canal. It is midline posteriorly mostly. It may be acute or chronic.

SAQ 6 What are the causes of anal incontinence?

- Perineal descent
- Malignancy irradiation
- Psychological
- Spina bifida
- Rectal prolapse
- Surgery
- Multiple sclerosis
- Old age
- Child birth
- Spinal injuries

SAQ 7 How a patient of fissure presents?

- Pain
- Bleeding
- Discharge

It has to be differentiated from Ca anus, proctalgia fugax, tuberculous ulcer, mitiple fissures of HIV.

LAQ 8 How to treat fissure in ano?

Conservative

- Glyceryl trinitrate cream
- Diltiazem
- Xylocaine cream
- Laxatives

Operative

- Dilating the anus
- Lateral anal sphincterotomy
- Anal advancement flap

SAQ 9 What is proctagia fugax?

It is a sudden cramp-like pain generally when the patient lies on bed, last for minutes and disappears spontaneously, recurring at irregular interval and without organic cause.

LAQ 10 What are haemorrhoids or piles?

Greek *Haima* = blood; *Rhoos* = flowing

These are dilated veins, in relation to the anus, originating in subepithelial plexus by the radicles of superior, middle and inferior rectal veins. It may be external covered by skin and internal bneath the mucous membrane or interno-external. Symptomatic haemorrhoids occur secondary to:

- Ca rectum
- Constipation
- Pregnancy
- Straining during micturition.

SAQ 11 What are the causes of haemorrhoids?

- Hereditary
- Anatomical peculiarities
- Constipation
- Diarrhoea or dysentery

SAQ 12 What are the positions of internal haemorrhoids?

When the patient in lithotomy position, it is 3, 7 and 11o'clock position.

SAQ 13 How a piles patient present?

(i) Painless fresh bleeding P/R, if uncomplicated
(ii) It may hang:
1st degree: No mucosal prolapse
2nd degree: Mucosal prolapse during defaecation and reduced spontaneously
3rd degree: Prolapse is reduced manually
4th degree: It is always prolapsed

SAQ 14 What are the complications of piles?

- Strangulation
- Ulceration
- Infection
- Portal pyaemia
- Bleeding
- Thrombosis
- Gangrene
- Pyelophlebitis
- Fibrosis

LAQ 15 How to treat bleeding piles?

Symptomatic treatment with isogel or proprietary creams.

Active treatment:

(i) Injection of sclerosing agent 5% phenol in almond oil or arachis oil
(ii) Banding
(iii) Photocoagulation
(iv) Haemorrhoidectomy (open, closed technique or endostapling technique)

SAQ 16 What postoperative complications may arise out of piles operation?

Early: • Pain • Retention of urine • Reactionary haemorrhage
Late: • Secondary haemorrhage • Anal stricture • Fissure incontinence.

SAQ 17 What are the causes of pruritus ani?

Intractable itching around anus (Pruritus ani) may occur with:

- Lack of cleanliness, woolen underclothes
- Vaginal discharge
- Epidermophytosis
- Skin disease
- Perianal discharge
- Parasitic
- Allergy
- Psychoneurosis

SAQ 18 What do mean by partial and complete prolapse of rectum?

In partial prolapse: Mucus membrane and submucosa of the rectum protrude outside the anus up to 1.25–3.75 cm composed of no more than double layers.

In complete prolapse (procidentia): It is more than 3.75 cm and it is thicker and double the thickness of entire rectum. Any prolapse more than 5 cm contains a layer of peritoneum.

LAQ 19 What are the different methods of treatment of prolapse rectum?

Treatment of prolapse rectum

- **Young age**
  - Partial
    - Digital reposition
    - Submucosal injection of 5% phenol in almond oil
  - Complete
    - Thiersch operation
- **Old age**
  - Submucosal injection
  - Excision of partial prolapse and Goodsall ligature (if unilateral)
  - Thiersch operation
  - Operative suspension of prolapsed bowel
  - Weil's operation (rectum is fixed to sacrum by polyvinyl alcohol sponge)
  - Ripstain operation (rectosegmoid junction is hitched up by teflon sling)
  - Lahauts operation: Mobilising rectum and sigmoid colon and holding it by rectus sheath

SAQ 20 Classify ano-rectal abscess.

Anorectal abscess

- Perianal (60%)
- Ischeorectal (30%)
- Submucus (5%)
- Pelvirectal
- Fissure abscess

SAQ 21 What is fistula in ano?

It is track lined by granulation tissue opening into rectum or anal canal deeply and skin around rectum superficially. It may be ***high level*** if opens above anorectal ring and ***low level*** if opens below anorectal ring.

SAQ 22 What is Goodsall rule?

Fistulae with external opening relation to anterior half of anus tend to be straight direct type and with external opening relation to posterior half have a curve track.

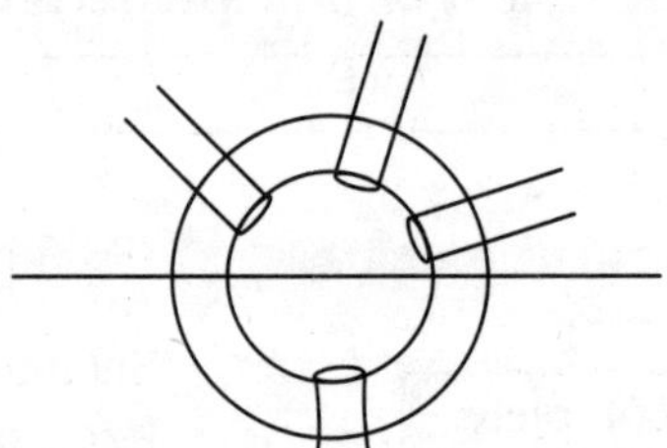

SAQ 23 Name the different investigations of fistula in ano.

(a) Digital examination
(b) Proctoscopy
(c) Probing
(d) Radiology of chest to rule out Tb and sinus with lipiodl or other opaque medium. Endoluminal USG and MRI

SAQ 24 How will you treat fistula in ano?

By excision of the fistula. Unhealthy granulation tissue is scrapped by Volkmann's spoon or the whole fibrous linning is excised. Biopsy of the fistula should be send always.

SAQ 25 Name some conditions producing benign anal stricture and how it is treated.

Benign anal stricture

- **Congenital**
- **Spasmodic**
  - In fissure
- **Organic**
  - Postoperative
  - Irradiation
  - Senile
  - Lymphogranuloma inguinale
  - Crohn's disease
  - Endometriosis

Treatment

(i) Anal dilatation by bougies or dilator
(ii) Anoplasty
(iii) Colostomy
(iv) Rectal excision and coloanal anastomosis

LAQ 26 Name the different polyps of the rectum.

Polyp rectum

- Hamartoma
  - Juvenile polyp
  - Peutz-Jeghers syndrome
- Neoplastic
  - Adenoma
  - Villous papilloma
- Inflammatory
  - Ulcerative colitis
  - Crohn's disease
- Metaplastic
  - Familial Polyposis

LAQ 27 Name the different malignant lesions of the anus and anal cancer.

- Squmous cell carcinoma
- Basaloid carcinoma or clonogenic carcinoma
- Mucoepidermoid carcinoma
- Basal cell carcinoma
- Melanoma
- Lymphoma
- Bowen's disease
- Paget's disease
- Kaposi's tumour

SAQ 28 What are the different methods of treatment of anal cancer?

(i) Local excision leaving a margin of 2.5 cm tissue all around
(ii) Abdominoperitoneal resection
(iii) Radiotherapy
(iv) Chemotherapy,

LAQ 29 How the anal intraepithelial neoplasms (AIN) are classified?

Classification of AIN:

AIN I: Cellular and nuclear abnormalities restricted to lower one-third of the epithelium
AIN II: Lower two-thirds of epithelium are affected
AIN III: Full thickness of epithelium are affected

AIN is linked to human papilloma virus 16 and 18, common in female with systemic immuno-compromise.

AIN III is high malignant, the different modalities of treatment are:

- Excision
- Excision and grafting
- Laser
- Cryoablation
- Cytotoxic cream (5FU)

29 Hernia and Umbilicus

SAQ 1 Define hernia.

It is protrusion of a viscus or a part of it through an abnormal opening in the walls of its containing cavity, viz.

- Epigastric
- Divarication recti
- Femoral
- Gluteal
- Paraumbilical
- Inguinal
- Obturator superior and inferior lumbar
- Sciatic

SAQ 2 What are causes of abdominal hernia?

- Raised intraabdominal pressure (viz. coughing, straining)
- Obesity
- Pregnancy
- Intraabdominal malignancy.

SAQ 3 What are the types of hernia?

(i) **Reducible:** Hernial contents can be returned back to intestine. For intestine, first portion is difficult to reduce and for omentum last portion is difficult to reduce.
(ii) **Irreducible:** Contents cannot be returned to abdomen without other complications
(iii) **Obstructed:** Irreducible hernia containg intestine, is obstructed from within or without
(iv) **Strangulated:** Blood supply of the contents is seriously impaired causing ischaemia or gangrene.
(v) **Incarcerated hernia:** Here lumen of the hernial sac is blocked by faeces.
(vi) **Ritcher's hernia:** In Ritcher's hernia, the hernial sac contains a portion of circumference of gut luman.
(vii) **Inflamed hernia:** Contents sec is inflamed from inflamed appendix or salpingitis.

LAQ 4 Describe in brief the anatomy of inguinal canal.

Extent: Extends from deep inguinal ring to superficial inguinal ring which are opening in fascia transversalis and external oblique aponeurosis, respectively.

Boundary: **Anteriorly**: External oblique aponeurosis in whole length, internal oblique, superficial fascia and skin

Posterioly: By fascia transversalis and medial aspect by conjoined tendon.

Roof: Internal oblique and transversus abdominis
Floor: By inguinal ligament
Contents:
(i) Spermatic cord in male or round ligament of uterus in female
(ii) Ilioinguinal nerve
(iii) Iliohypogastric nerve.

SAQ 5 What is Hesselbach's triangle?

This triangle is bounded medially by lateral border of rectus muscle, laterally by inferior epigastric artery and below by medial part of inguinal ligament. Through this weak point direct, inguinal hernia protrude.

LAQ 6 What are the different varieties of inguinal hernia?

A. According to extent

- **Incomplete**: Not entered scrotum
- **Complete**: Entered the scrotum

B. According to nature

Congenital or acquired

C. According to contents

Enterocele (intestine); omentocele (omentum); cytocele (bladder)

D. According to site of protrusion

- **Indirect**: Comes through deep inguinal ring. It may be bubonocele limited to scrotum funicular up to testis; vaginal whole length of processus and hernia descends down the scrotum.
- **Direct**: It comes out through Hesselbach's triangle.

LAQ 7 What are the differences between indirect and drect inguinal hernia?

	Indirect	Direct
Anatomical	Hernial neck is lateral to inferior epigastric artery, required skillful separation of spermatic cord. Neck is the narrowest part.	Lies medial to inferior epigastric artery. Sac is not attached to cord and sac is wide
Clinical	• Occurs in any age • More in males • Usually unilateral • Usually complete • Descends obliquely down and medially • Coughing impulse is felt on tip • Hernia fails to appear in deep ring occlusion test	• Rare before 40 • Almost rare in female • Usually bilateral • Usually incomplete • Forward bulge • Coughing impulse felt on pulp • It appears even after deep ring occlusion test.

SAQ 8 What is Maydl's hernia and Littre's hernia?

Maydl's hernia: Successive loops of bowel come in sacs, comes back in abdomen and re-enter sac like M or W pattern.

Littre's hernia: Hernial sac contents, Meckel's diverticulum.

SAQ 9 How to treat hernia?

Operation is the only treatment for hernia (Open; or laparoscopic)

Different operations are:

(i) Herniotomy
(ii) Herniorrhaphy (repair of inguinal canal Bassini's operation)
(iii) Hernioplasty (reinforcement of inguinal canal)
(iv) Laparoscopic herniorrhaphy by transperitoneal or transabdominal approach

SAQ 10 What is dual or saddle or Pantaloon hernia?

Here hernia consists of two sacs which straddle the inferior epigastric artery laterally and medially.

SAQ 11 What are the peculiarities of femoral hernia?

(i) More in female
(ii) Truss cannot control it
(iii) Stragulation is common, so should be operated as early as possible.

SAQ 12 What are the causes of recurrence of hernia?

Hernial recurrence

Faults in patient
- Weak muscle
- Cough
- Constipation
- Use of prolong truss

Faults in hernia
- Direct
- Large sliding

Faults in operation
- Postoperation infection

SAQ 13 What is the boundary of femoral canal?

Medially: Lacunar ligament

Laterally: By femoral vein with thin septum

Anteriorly: Inguinal ligament

Posteriorly: Fascia over pectineus muscle and ligament of Cooper.

SAQ 14 What are the different operations done for femoral hernia?

Different opproaches to treat femoral hernia are from:

(i) Above the inguinal ligament (Lotheissen's operation)
(ii) From below the inguinal ligament (Lockwood operation)
(iii) From above and below the inguinal ligament (McEvedy' operation)

SAQ 15 What is exomphalos?

Exomphalos or omphalocele or umbilical hernia occurs in 1:6000 birth due to failure of part of the midgut to return to coelom in fetal life. When the sac is unruptured, it contains outer amniotic membrane and inner peritoneum. If it is more than 4 cm, it is herniation of umbilical cord. Smaller defects are called umbilo-enteric fistula.

SAQ 16 What is paraumbilical hernia?

This type of hernia occurs through weak spot in linea alba either above (supraumbilical) or below (infraumbilical).

LAQ 17 How to treat umbilical hernia?

A. **Conservative**: Apply antiseptic solution so that granulation tissue from periphery rapair the later
B. Skin operative flap closure
C. Staged closure with prosthetic material
D. Paraumbilical hernia is treated by:
   (i) Epigastric herniorrhaphy
   (ii) Paraumbilical hernioplasty
   (iii) Additional lipectomy
   (iv) Mayo's operation

SAQ 18 What is divarication of recti?

Here there is wide gap between two rectus abominis muscles, through which abdominal contents bulge out.

SAQ 19 What are the types of perineal hernia?

This rare type of hernia may be:

(i) Postoperative
(ii) Median sliding perineal
(iii) Anterolateral perineal
(iv) Posterolateral perineal

SAQ 20 What is omphalitis? What complications it can produce?

It is infection of the umbilicus.

Complications:

- Abscess of abdominal wall with extensive ulceration
- Septicaemia
- Jaundice in newborn
- Portal vein thrombosis and portal hypertension
- Peritonitis
- Hernia

SAQ 21 What is umbilical granuloma?

Chronic infection of the umbilical cicatrix for several weeks produces umbilical granuloma treated by application of silver nitrate.

SAQ 22 What is umbolith or umbilical calculus?

Umbilical calculus is composed of desquamated epithelium, becomes inspissated and collected in umbilicus. Generally, it is black in colour. It is treated by dilating the orifice and to extract the calculus. For recurrence, excision of umbilicus is done.

SAQ 23 Name the different remnants of vitello intestinal duct.

(i) Umbilical fistula
(ii) Intraabdominal cyst
(iii) Intraperitoneal band
(iv) Meckel's diverticulum with a band adherent.

It should be excised together with Meckel's diverticulum preferably when the child is 6 months of age.

SAQ 24 Name the different neoplasm of umbilicus.

(i) **Benign:** Umbilical adenoma or respberry tumour; endometrioma
(ii) **Malignant:** Secondary (Sister Joseph nodule primary in stomach, colon or ovary)

LAQ 25 What is abdominal dehiscence?

Abdominal wound may brust in 6–8 days after operation and viscera is extruded. Causes are:

(i) Poor closure technique
(ii) Deep wound infection
(iii) Cough or vomiting
(iv) Poor general condition of patient (viz. obesity, jaundice, malignancy, hypoproteinaemia)

Protruding organ and omentum is washed gently with saline and returned to abdominal cavity and abdomen is sutured by monofilament nylon passed enough plastic rubber collar. It is an emergency operation.

SAQ 26 Name some neoplasms of abdominal wall.

- Desmoid tumour (from musculoaponeurotic structures of abdominal wall)
- Fibrosarcoma
- Adenocarcinoma

Urinary Symptoms: Anuria, Kidney

30

LAQ 1 What is haematuria? What are its important etiologies?

Haematuria is presence of blood in urine (microscopic, detected by dipstick test or macroscopic). It is always abnormal. It may be intermittent or persistant. Important causes of haematuria are:

1. **Blood dyscrasia:** Purpura, anticoagulant, sickle cell trait.
2. **Tumours:** Transitional cell Ca; Wilms' tumour, hypernephroma, urethral and ureter neoplasm
3. **Kidney:** Infarct, injury; Tb, nephritis, stone
4. **Bladder:** Tb; cystitis,tumour, stone, Bilharzia
5. **Prostate:** Enlargement (benign or malignant)

LAQ 2 What are the important symptoms of urinary tract?

(1) Haematuria (2) Pain

Upper urinary tract	Lower urinary tract
Deep fixed, brusting, colicky, may referred to groin, scrotum or labium	Suprapubic discomfort, burning in character may be referred to tip of the penis

Altered bladder function: As urgency, hesitancy, pis-en deux (patient tries to micturate even after it is completed), chronic retention with overflow.

LAQ 3 Name the important investigations of urinary tract.

1. Urinalysis (microscopic, cytological, biochemical, bacteriological)
2. Renal function test (blood urea, creatinine, cromium 51 labelled ethylenediamine tetra-acetic acid clearance).
3. Imaging
   - KUB
   - Intravenous urography
   - Retrograde ureterogram
   - Antegrade pyelogram
   - USG and transrectal USG
   - Digital subtraction arteriography
4. Cystography
5. Ureterography
6. Venography
7. CT
8. MRI
9. PET
10. Radioisotope scan
11. Endoscope (by Nitze's cystoscope)

SAQ 4 Define oliguria and anuria.

Oliguria is less than 300 ml of urine day. Anuria is complete absence of urine.

LAQ 5 What are important causes of renal failure?

Renal failure causes

Prerenal causes

- Hypovolemia
- Haemorrhage
- Sepsis
- Cardiogenic
- Shock
- Anaesthesia
- Hypoxia

Renal causes

- Drugs
- Poisons
- Contrast media
- Eclampsia
- Myoglobinuria
- Incompatible blood transfusion
- DIC

Obstructive or postrenal causes

- Stone
- Malignancy
- Surgery
- Bilharziasis
- Retroperitoneal fibrosis
- Crystaluria

SAQ 6 What are the different methods of treating obstructive renal failure?

(i) Catheterization (urethral or suprapubic)
(ii) Indwelling stents
(iii) Percutaneous nephrostomy
(iv) Open surgery

SAQ 7 How are the kidneys developed?

Wolffian duct goes backwards behind peritoneum from which ureter and renal pelvis develops. Metanephros produces renal parenchyma. Continuity of glomerular apparatus and nephrotic tubules is formed. Each kidney ascends to original position and hilum rotates medially from forwards.

SAQ 8 What are congenital abnormalities of kidney and ureter?

(i) Absence of kidney
(ii) Renal ectopia (kidney remains in pelvis)
(iii) Horseshoe-shaped kidney
(iv) Unilateral s-fusion the kidney
(v) Polycystic kidney
(vi) Infantile polycystic disease
(vii) Unilateral multicystic disease
(viii) Solitary renal cyst
(ix) Abberent renal vessels
(x) Duplication of renal pelvis
(xi) Duplication of a ureter
(xii) Megaureter (congenital)
(xiii) Postcaval ureter
(xiv) Ureterocele.

LAQ 9 Write short note on polycystic kidney.

It arises due to failure of fusion between secretory and excretory parts of the developing kidney. Usually mesonephric cap fuses with metanephros and if there is failure of fusion between the two, then secretory part gets dilated to produce multiple cyst. The tubules develop in different zones at different times, usually one disappear and other appear.

The cut section of the kidney specimen shows:

(a) Multiple cyst showing honeycomb appearance with intervening healthy parenchyma,
(b) Some of the surface is bossilated

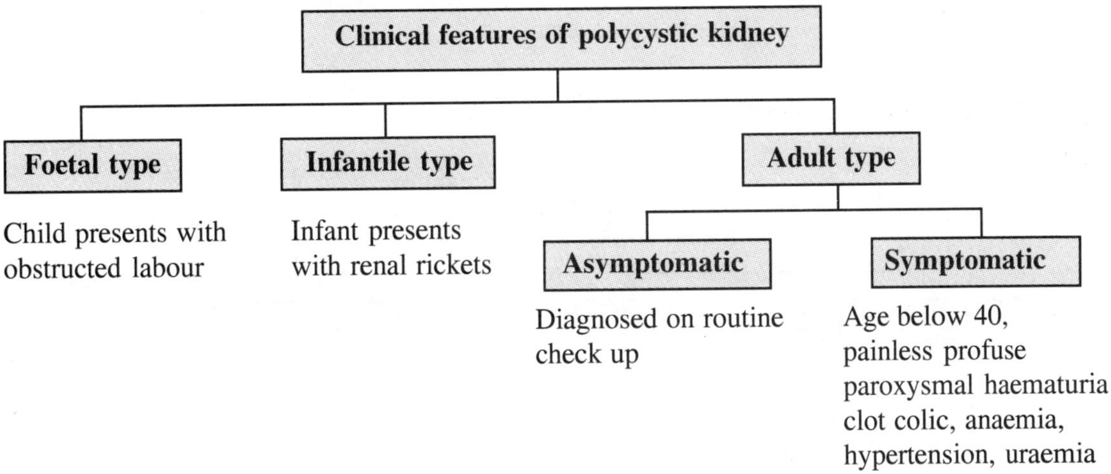

Investigations: History; physical exam, blood Hb; urine sp gr low, X-ray (enlarged kidney: USG, IVP; retrograde pyelogram (spider leg appearance), cystoscopy; chromocystoscopy (indicocaramine 7.5 ml).

Treatment

(a) **Conservative:** More fluid, less protein, haematinics, anabolic steroids, antibiotics; ask the patient to avoid crowded place
(b) **Surgery-Rovsing operation:** Puncture as many cysts as possible in single sitting to relief pressure effect of enlarged cyst to healthy parenchyma.

SAQ 10 Name some other cystic conditions.

There are many, but the important are pancreatic, lung, breast, etc.

SAQ 11 What is hydronephrosis?

It is the aseptic dilatation of pelvicallicial system due to long continued obstruction of urinary outflow. It may be:

(i) Congenital or acquired
(ii) Unilateral or bilateral
(iii) Pelvic type, renal type or pelvi-renal type.

SAQ 12 What is the mechanism of unilateral and bilateral hydronephrosis?

Any obstruction proximal to the bladder will cause unilateral hydronephrosis and any obstruction in or below bladder will cause bilateral hydronephrosis.

LAQ 13 Enumerate the causes of hydronephrosis.

Hydronephrosis causes

Unilateral

Extramural:
- Adjacent tumour
- Retrocaval ureter
- Retroperitoneal fibrosis

Mural:
- Calculus
- Papillary necrosis
- Analgesic abusers

Intramural:
- Neoplasm of ureter
- Tb
- Calculus
- Stenosis

Bilateral

Congenital
- Stricture meatus
- Phimosis
- Valves in urethra
- Bladder neck stricture

Acquired
- BPH
- Ca prostates
- Neck obstruction
- Phimosis
- Urethral stricture

SAQ 14 Describe the pathology of hydronephrosis.

The whole of the kidney is stretched and kidney parenchyma is atrophied. Cut section of the kidney shows multiple cavities lined by stretched out renal parenchyma. Some of them may show presence of stone. In pelvic type, only pelvis of kidney is distended with least effect on parenchyma.

SAQ 15 How will you investigate a case of hydronephrosis?

- Urine RE/CS
- X-ray KUB
- USG
- Blood Hb
- IVP
- Urea and NPN
- Retrograde pyelogram

SAQ 16 How a hydronephrosis patient present?

- Pain loin (coliky or dull aching)
- Kidney lump (uni- or bilateral lump may disappear with passage of large amount ofurine if it is intermittent).
- Haematuria
- Infection
- Impairment of kidney functions.

SAQ 17 How will you treat hydronephrosis?

Control infection and assess renal function before surgery.

Nephrectomy: If the kidney is grossly affected and other kidney is completely functioning.

Nephrolithotomy or pyelolithotomy: If cause is stone.

Pyeloplasty (Anderson-Hynes disjunction pyeloplasty)

Endoscopic pyelolysis: Desruption of pelvi-ureteric junction by balloon distension.

LAQ 18 What are the causes of renal stone?

Important causes of renal stone are:

(i) Dietetic (deficient vitamin A)
(ii) Altered urinary solutes and colloids (dehydration, decreased citrate)
(iii) Urine stasis
(iv) Renal infection
(v) Immobilisation causing decalcification of skeleton
(vi) Hyperparathyroid state
(vii) Erosion of renal papilla (Randall's plaque)

SAQ 19 What are the important types of renal stones?

Renal stone types:

(i) Oxalate stone
(ii) Phosphate stone in UTI by *Proteus*
(iii) Uric acid stone
(iv) Cystine stone (hexagonal crystal)
(v) Xanthine stone (round brick colour with lamellation)

SAQ 20 How a renal stone patient presents?

(i) Silent
(ii) Pain (fixed to renal angle or ureteric colic)
(iii) Haematuria
(iv) Pyuria
(iv) During colic attack, there may be rigidity of lateral abdominal muscle

SAQ 21 How to investigate renal stone?

- KUB X-ray
- Excretion urography
- USG
- Spiral CT

SAQ 22 What are the different methods of treatment for renal stone?

(a) (i) Conservative treatment if the stone is less than 0.5 mm and not impacted as because it may pass spontaneously. Following surgery may be done after controlling infection.
(ii) Percutaneous nephrolithotomy
(iii) Extracorporeal shock wave lithotripsy

(b) **Open surgery for renal stones:**
(i) Pyelolithotomy
(ii) Extended pyelolithotomy
(iii) Nephrolithotomy

(c) If both the kidneys are affected with stone, the better functioning kidney's stone is removed first

SAQ 23 What is Brodel's line?

It is relatively avascular area in the kidney where anterior and posterior branches of renal artery meet, preferred for site of renal incision.

SAQ 24 What are the different anatomical narrowing in ureter?

(i) Ureteropelvic junction
(ii) Site of iliac artery crossing it
(iii) Crossing of vas deferens or broad ligament
(iv) Where entering bladder and
(v) At ureteric orifice

LAQ 25 What are the different treatments for ureteric colic?

For pain NSAID. Surgical removal is required if:

(i) Stone is enlarging and obstructing kidney
(ii) UTI
(iii) Large stone
(iv) Repeated pain but stone is stagnant
(v) Solitary kidney stone or bilateral large stone

Stones may be removed by:

(a) Closed method
- (i) Dormia basket
- (ii) Ureteroscope
- (iii) Push bang ureteric stone is pushed back by catheter, repositioned by J-stent and removed by **E**xtracorporeal **S**hock **W**ave **L**ithotripsy (ESWL)

(b) Open method
- (i) Ureterolithotomy

SAQ 26 How is the kidney infected?

It may receive infection from haematogenous spread or by ascending infection.

SAQ 27 What is pyonephrosis?

Here kidney is converted to multilocular sac containing pus or purulent urine. After diagnosing, perenteral antibiotics are given and pus is drained, if required by nephrostomy (percutaneous or open). Nephrectomy is required if kidney is damaged.

SAQ 28 What are the causes of perinephric abscess?

(i) Perirenal haematoma
(ii) Tuberculous vertebra
(iii) Extension from cortical abscess
(iv) Infected appendix
(v) Blood brought
(vi) Via urethral lymphatics

LAQ 29 Describe in brief the pathogenesis of renal tuberculosis.

It is always secondary to primary focus which is often impossible to identify, via haematogenous or lymphatics spread, settles at the apex of renal papilla of renal pyramid producing tubercle formation. The different pathological types are:

(i) Caseous type
(ii) Cavernous type
(iii) Caseo-cavernous type
(iv) Ulcerative type
(v) Hydronephrotic type
(vi) Fibrous type (rare)
(vii) Pyonephrosis
(viii) Putty kidney

Renal Tb should be a suspicion, if:

(i) Cystis even after antibiotics
(ii) Sterile pyuria
(iii) Obstructive lesion throughout urinary tract
(iv) Chronic inflammation and scarring

SAQ 30 How renal tuberculosis patient presents?

(i) **General features of TB**
(ii) **Local features:** • Frequency • Painless haematuria • Features of cystitis • Loin pain.

SAQ 31 What are the causes of frequency of micturition in genitourinary tuberculosis?

(i) Tuberculous bacilluria causing irritation
(ii) Passage of debris through urine
(iii) Tuberculous cystitis
(iv) Contracted or systolic bladder

SAQ 32 What are the different surgical treatments of renal tuberculosis?

It should be done if ATD fails to eradicate the lesion. Different surgeries are:

(a) Cavernostomy
(b) Partial nephrectomy if lesion in lower lobe
(c) Nephrectomy—when one kidney is completely damaged and other kidney is healthy.

SAQ 33 Name some renal neoplasm.

Renal neoplasms

Benign

- Adenoma
- Angioma
- Angiomyolipoma

Malignant

- Wilms' tumour
- Hypernephroma
- Papillary transitional cell Ca of renal pelvis
- Squamous cell Ca of renal pelvis

LAQ 34 Write short note on Wilms' tumour.

(i) Mixed tumour containing embryonic nephrogenic tissue of epithelial and connective tissue, bone, cartilage or muscle
(ii) Usually presents before 4 years in one pole of kidney
(iii) Presents with pyrexia and haematuria
(iv) Cut surface of tumour is pinkish or grayish white.
(v) Diagnosed by USG, CT
(vi) Metastatise to lung via blood
(vii) Treated by **nephrectomy** at earliest followed by **radiotherapy** with or without **chemotherapy**. If both kidneys are affected, partial nephrectomy

LAQ 35 What is hypernephroma/adenocarcinoma of kidney/Garwitz tumours? How it presents?

This arises from renal tubular cells, moderate size tumour generally on upper pole.

Cut surface is yellow or dull white, semitransparent with haemorrhage, devided into lobule by septa. **Microscopically** with solid polyhedral cells deeply staining with round nuclei and abundant cytoplasm with lipid cholesterol and glycogen.

Spreads by vein and produces cannon ball secondary deposits. It also spread by lymphatics. It is common in men **presents** with clot colic, loin discomfort and mass or with metastatic presentation (viz. pathological fracture, haemoptosis); fever, anemia or polycythaemia, raised ESR or nephrotic syndrome.

SAQ 36 How is hypernephroma diagnosed?

- IVU
- Renal angiography
- USG
- CXR (PA)
- CT with enhancement

SAQ 37 How is hypernephroma treated?

It is treated by nephrectomy. Vascular pedicle should be ligated first to avoid metastasis. Cytokine and interleukin-2 shows promising result, but radiotherapy or chemotherapy are not that effective.

SAQ 38 Name some conditions where nephrectomy is done for benign conditions.

(i) Atrophic or dysplastic kidney
(ii) Accelerated hypertension

31 Urinary Bladder

SAQ 1 How the urinary bladder is innervated?

Sympathetic: 11th thoracic to second lumbar fibre via presacral hypogastric nerve via sympathetic chain to inferior hypogastric plexus.

Parasympathetic: S_2–S_4 via pelvic splanchnic nerve to inferior hypogastric to bladder.

Somatic: Pudendal nerves

SAQ 2 What is ectopia vesicae or exstrophy of the bladder?

This congenital condition is characterised by incomplete development of anterior abdominal wall (infraumbilical) and anterior urinary bladder wall development.

Edges of abdominal wall can be felt; umbilicus is absent.

Treated with iliac osteostomy (1st year), followed by closure of bladder and anterior abdominal wall. Reconstruction of bladder neck and sphincter may be required.

LAQ 3 What are the important causes of retention of urine?

Retention of urine may be acute, chronic or chronic with overflow:

Retention of urine causes

In male

- Urethral strictures
- Postoperative
- Bladder outlet obstruction
- Phimosis
- Prostate enlargement

In female

- Retroverted pregnant uterus
- Multiple sclerosis

In both male and female

- Clot or calculus
- Rupture urethra
- Faecal impaction
- Spinal anaesthesia

Retention of urine presents with:

(i) No urine for several hours
(ii) Visible tender bladder which is dull on percussion

LAQ 4 How to diagnose urinary incontinence?

(i) History, physical examination, voiding chart
(ii) Urodynamic testing
(iii) Urine culture
(iv) Serum creatinine
(v) IVU

Urodynamic testing helps to differentiate:

(a) Incontinence
(b) Neurogenic bladder
(c) Stress incontinence
(d) Bladder outflow obstruction

Some causes of incontinence:

- Alzheimer
- Neurogenic bladder
- Fistulae
- Parkinsonism
- Weak sphincter
- Cerebral infarct
- Tuberculosis of bladder

LAQ 5 Write short note on bladder stone.

Types

(i) **Primary**: Develops in sterile urine, originates in kidney passes down to bladder.
(ii) **Scondary** bladder stone develops in infected urine.

It may be: (a) oxalate, (b) uric acid stone, (c) cystine stone, (d) phosphate stone

Clinical presentation

- Pain (tip of penis in male in labia majora in female) and strangury.
- Haematuria
- Frequency or interruption of urine stream

Treatment

- Litholapaxy (not done if there is stricture or stone is large)
- Suprapubic lithotomy
- Percutaneous suprapubic litholapaxy
- **E**xtracorporeal **S**hock **W**ave **L**ithotripsy (ESWL)

LAQ 6 What are the causes of diverticulum of bladder? What complications it may produce? How is it diagnosed and treated?

A bladder diverticulum may be:

(i) Congenital or
(ii) Pulsion diverticulum due to outflow obstruction

Complications:

• Urinary infection • Bladder stone • Hydronephrosis • Neoplasm

Diagnosed by:

(i) Cystoscopy (ii) IVU (iii) USG (iv) Retrograde cystography

Bladder diverticulum is treated by operation if there is complication.

SAQ 7 What is hernia of bladder or traction diverticulum?

Here a portion of bladder protrudes through inguinal or femoral hernial orifice.

LAQ 8 What is fistula? What are causes of urinary fistula?

Fistula is a communication between two epithelial lined surfaces. Urinary fistula may be: (i) intraperitoneal, (ii) extraperitoneal, (iii) paraperitoneal

Causes: (i) Congenital, (ii) traumatic

Varieties: • Vesicovaginal • Fistula from renal pelvis to skin or gut in Tb • Fistula from infection as in Crohn's disease • Fistula due to carcinoma (bladder or bowel) • Urethral fistula (stricture, rupture, etc.)

LAQ 9 What is cystitis? What are the causes of bladder infection?

Cystitis is inflammation of bladder mostly due to infection.

It may be due to ascending infection, urethral instrumentation, from neighbouring structure, descending infection

Predisposing factors are:

- Incomplete emptying
- Diabetes mellitus
- Immune suppression
- Calculus, neoplasm, foreign body
- Oestrogen deficiency

SAQ 10 How a cystitis patient presents?

- Urinary frequency
- Suprapubic pain
- Haematuria
- Pyuria

SAQ 11 What complications may arise out of urethral catheterization?

- Urethritis
- Cystitis
- Epididymitis
- Prostatitis
- Orchitis
- Pyelonephritis

SAQ 12 What is Hunner's ulcer or interstitial cystitis?

It is pancystitis with infiltration of lymphocyte and macrophages causing fibrosis, contracture of bladder and avascular atrophy of the epithelium, ulceration of bladder fundus mostly in woman causing distress.

SAQ 13 What is alkaline encrusting cystitis?

Here urea splitting organism causes phosphate encrustation of bladder, treated by removing encrustation by bladder irrigation and appropriate antibiotics.

SAQ 14 What is cystitis cystica?

(i) Bladder mucosa is deficient of glands.
(ii) Over trigone surface epithelium sends of buds causing cysts with clear fluids
(iii) Adenocarcinoma may arise

SAQ 15 How schistosomiasis of bladder is diagnosed?

(i) Examination of urine (ELISA or MAMA, i.e. *S. mansoni* adult microsound antigen)
(ii) Cystoscopy may show (Bilharzial pseudotubercle, sandy patches, ulceration, fibrosis, granuloma papilloma, carcinoma)

SAQ 16 Name the different occupational workers prone to bladder cancer.

The following occupational workers are prove to Ca bladder:

- Textile workers
- Dye
- Rubber tube
- Shoe manufacturer
- Chimney cleaner
- Lorry divers

SAQ 17 Name some carcinoma of bladder.

(i) Transitional cell carcinoma

(ii) In situ carninoma

(iii) Superficial bladder cancer (papillary tumour with exophytic growth fashion in bladder lumen)

(iv) Muscle invasive transitional cell carcinoma

(v) Squamous cell carcinoma

(vi) Adenocarcinoma

SAQ 18 How to investigate bladder carcinoma?

(i) Bimannual exam

(ii) Examination of urine (**N**uclear **M**atrix **P**roteins NMP22 for recurrent tumours)

(iii) IVU

(iv) Cystourethroscopy

LAQ 19 How to treat carcinoma of bladder?

Treatment of Ca bladder

Non-invasive variety

(i) Endoscopic surgery
(ii) Intravesicle chemotherapy thiotepa, mitomycin, epirubicin, doxorubicin or immunotherapy (BCG)
(iii) Open surgical excision

Invasive variety

(i) Radiotherapy (Deep external beam X-ray or local radiotherapy)
(ii) Surgery (partial cystectomy; and pelvic lymphodenectomy)

SAQ 20 What is Leukoplakia of bladder?

Here there is squamous metaplasia of the bladder with production of keratin and passage of white particles in urine. Localised leukoplakia resected endoscopically. Diffuse leukoplakia is premalignant and require cystectomy.

LAQ 21 What are the indications of urinary diversion?

Following are the indications of urinary diversion:

Urinary diversion

- **Temporary**
  - To relieve temporary obstruction
- **Permanent**
  - Bladder removed
  - Incurable fistula
  - Neurological defect of bladder

LAQ 22 What are the different methods of urinary diversion?

Methods of urinary diversion

- **Temporary**
  - Foley catheter
  - Double 'J' ureteric pigtail stents
- **Permanent**
  - **External division**
    - Ileal conduit
  - **Internal division**
    - To colon and rectum
    - Bladder reconstruction
    - Continent urinary diversion
    - Bladder substitution augmentation

SAQ 23 What are the complications of internal urinary diversion?

- Stricture
- Resorption of solutes
- Urinary reflux
- Risk of cancer.

32 Prostate and Seminal Vesicles

SAQ 1 What are different zones of prostate glands?

According to McNeal prostate has:

(i) Peripheral zone (ii) Central zone (iii) Periurethral transitional zone

LAQ 2 Describe the surgical anatomy of prostate.

This fibromuscular glandular organ in the shape of chest nut, situated below bladder, in front of rectum, above urogenital diaphragm and behind symphysis pubis anteriorly. It has following lobes:

(i) Anterior lobe in front of urethra made up of fibrous tissue
(ii) Two lateral lobes
(iii) One posterior lobe
(iv) One median lobe situated above the prostate utricle and in between ejaculatory ducts.

Following are the important prostate contents inside out:

(i) Urethral gands
(ii) Intermediate submucous glands also known as adenomatous zone
(iii) Outermost subcapsular zone called carcinomatous zone.

SAQ 3 Write short note on PSA.

Prostate specific antigen (PSA) is glycoprotein, serine protease. It helps liquification of semen and acts as marker of prostatic diseases. Its value increases in Ca prostate <15 ng/ml (normal is 4 ng/ml), but it does not help in the differential diagnosis of BPH and Ca prostate (value 12 ng/ml).

SAQ 4 What are the etiologies of BPH?

Different etiologies are:

(i) Hormonal influence: Increase oestrogenic and intermediate peptide growth factor; and
(ii) Decreased serum testosterone.

LAQ 5 What are the effects of BPH?

Effects on urethra:
- Narrowed
- Elongated
- Tortuous because of intraureteric projection of prostate.

Bladder:
- Hypertrophy
- Dilatation
- Cystitis
- Retroprostatic pouch
- Diverticulum (may be with stone)
- Bladder outflow obstruction by increasing smooth muscle tone (under control of alpha agonist)

Kidney and ureter:
- Hydroureter or hydronephrosis
- Pyonephrosis
- Renal failure

SAQ 6 What is bladder outflow obstruction? What are the causes of it?

This urodynamic concept means low flow rates with high voiding pressure. Etiologies are:
- BPH
- Ca prostate
- Bladder neck stenosis or hypertrophy
- Urethral stricture

SAQ 7 What are the important symptoms of lower urinary tract?

(i) Hesitancy
(ii) Poor flow
(iii) Stop and start
(iv) Dribbing
(v) Poor emptying
(vi) Retention
(vii) Frequency
(viii) Nocturia
(ix) Urgency
(x) Incontinence

SAQ 8 Why there is frequency of micturition in BPH?

- Prostatic urethra is pulled up into bladder and irritate it
- Relaxation of internal sphincter
- Cystitis
- Irritation of trigone by intravesicle projection

LAQ 9 How will you diagnose and investigate BPH?

(i) History
(ii) Examination of abdomen (retention)
(iii) Anaemia and signs of CRF

(iv) Rectal examination (residual urine and enlarge prostate)
(v) PSA
(vi) Flow rate measurement
(vii) Pressure flow urodynamic studies
(viii) Blood (for Hb, creatinine, electrolytes)
(ix) Urinalysis
(x) USG or IVP
(xi) Cystourethroscopy
(xii) Transrectal USG
(xiii) Marian sign positive.

LAQ 10 How to treat BPH?

Conservative

- Fluid and coffee restriction
- Apha blocker
- 5 alpha reductase inhibitors.

Surgery

TRUP is gold standard done for:

- Acute retention
- Chronic retention with renal impairment
- High residual volume and low flow rate
- Diverticulum
- Haemorrhage

Open prostatectomy for large glands.

LAQ 11 What are the different methods of open prostatectomy?

(i) Suprapubic transvesicle (Frayer's operation)
(ii) Retropubic (Millin)
(iii) Transurethral
(iv) Young's perineal

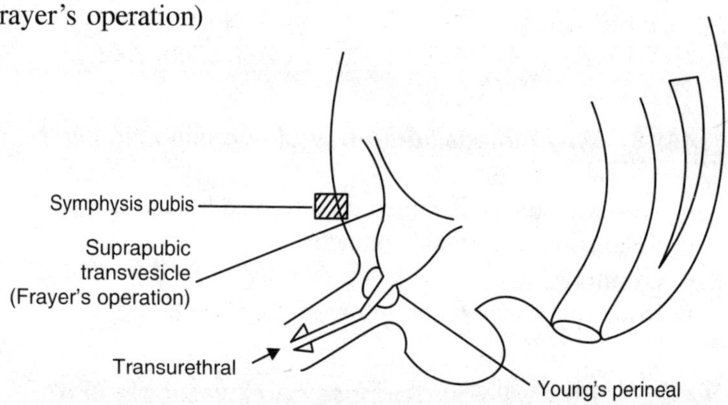

> Most urologist irrigate the bladder with three ways Folley catheter for 24 hours.

SAQ 12 What is corpora amylaceae?

Calcified laminated bodies in glandular prostate probably forerunner of endogenous prostatic calcula found in elderly males and apes.

LAQ 13 What are the complications of prostatectomy?

Complications

Local

- Haemorrhage
- Perforation of bladder
- Sepsis
- Incontinence
- Impotence
- Retrograde ejaculation
- Urethral stricture
- Bladder neck contracture
- Reoperation

General

- Water intoxication
- CVS
  (CCF; infarction, pneumonia, deep vein thrombosis)

LAQ 14 How the BPH and Ca prostate differs by P/R exam?

Patient is asked to lie left lateral or Genu elbow position and to take deep inspiration. Gloved finger is lubricated and gradually introduced into rectum.

	BPH	Ca Prostate
Size	Enlarged	Enlarged
Feel	Firm and elastic	Hard
Nodule	Nil	Present
Posterior groove	Deepened	Obliterated
Rectal m/membrane	Free and mobile	Fixed
Retroprostatic pouch	Well palpable	May not be appreciated

SAQ 15 Name some alpha blocking drugs with doses.

(i) Alfuzosin 2.5 mg BD or TDS
(ii) Doxazosin 1 mg at bedtime
(iii) Indoramin 20 mg BD
(iv) Prazosin 2 mg/day
(v) Terazosin 1 mg at night

SAQ 16 Describe the histological appearance of Ca prostate.

- Adenocarcinoma
- Glands appearing in confluence
- Loss of basement membrane
- Less differentiated as solid sheets

SAQ 17 How Ca prostate spreads?

(i) **Locally** to seminal vesicle, bladder neck, rectum, ureter
(ii) **Bloodstream** to bone, breast, kidney, bronchus, thyroid, femoral head
(iii) **Lymphatic** spreads to rectum, seminal vesicle, vas deferens, supraclavicular node

SAQ 18 How a Ca prostate patient presents?

- Bladder obstruction
- Pelvic pain
- Anemia or pancytopenia
- Features of BPH and nodule P/R
- Haematuria
- Malaise
- Kidney failures

SAQ 19 How Ca prostate is investigated?

Following tests are done for Ca prostate:

(i) Rectal examination
(ii) Biopsy of prostate
(iii) LFT, anaemia, urea, creatinine
(iv) PSA
(v) Acid phosphatase estimation
(vi) X-ray
(vii) USG
(viii) Bone scan
(ix) Lymphangiography
(xi) Bone marrow aspiration

LAQ 20 Mention the treatment of Ca prostate.

Treatment Ca prostate

Early stage

(i) Radical prostatectomy
(ii) Radiotherapy
  (a) **E**xternal **b**eam **r**adio **t**herapy (EBRT)
  (b) Brachytherapy

Advanced stage

(i) Orchidectomy
(ii) Medical castration
- Phosphorylated diethyl stilbesterol
- LHRH agonist
- Androgen receptor blocker (flutamide or bicalutamide cyproterone acetate)

(iii) General radiotherapy, IV strontium 89

LAQ 21 How acute and chronic prostitis presents and treated?

Presentation

Acute prostitis	Chronic prostitis
Fever Chill and rigor Dysuria Perianal heavyness Rectal irritation Defaecation	Perigenital pain Testicular pain Pain increases on intercourse Threads in urine Pus on prostatic massage
Treatment: Septran or ciprofloxacin	Septran; metronidazole, doxycycline

SAQ 22 What is prostatodynia?

Perigenital pain in absence of prostatic inflammation.

33 Urethra and Penis

SAQ 1 Name some congenital abnormalities of male urethra.

(i) Meatal stenosis
(ii) Urethral stricture
(iii) Duplication of urethra
(iv) Congenital valves
(v) Hypospadias (external meatus opens underside)
(vi) Epispadias (external meatus opens on dorsum)

LAQ 2 What are the different types of extravasation of urine? What are its treatment?

Extravasation of urine

	Superficial extravasation	Deep extravasation
Etiology	• Rupture bulbous urethra • False passage during urethral dilatation. • Refilling of bladder by repeated suprapubic puncture.	• Rupture membranous urethra • Extraperitoneal bladder rupture • Lower ureter injury.
Collection of urine	• Superficial perineal pouch; body of penis, anterior abdominal walls	• Collection of urine in perivesicle space
Clinical feature	History of trauma, gradual collection of urine, uriniferous smell, temperature	• History of trauma, retention of urine; mass in hypogastrium
Treatment	• Multiple incision on scrotum or penis to drain away collected fluid; antibiotic suprapublic cystostomy	• Suprapubic cystostomy followed by treatment of special injuries (ureter; urethra)

SAQ 3 What are the complications of rupture membranous urethra?

- Stricture
- Impotence
- Incontinance
- Extravasation of urine

SAQ 4 What are the causes of urethral stricture?

It may be:

(i) Congenital
(ii) Inflammatory (post-gonococcal, traumatic; cystoscopy or catheter)
(iii) Open prostatectomy
(iv) Amputation of penis

SAQ 5 What are the complications of urethral stricture?

- Urine retention
- Periurethral abscess
- Diverticulum or fistula

LAQ 6 What are the different treatments of urethral stricture?

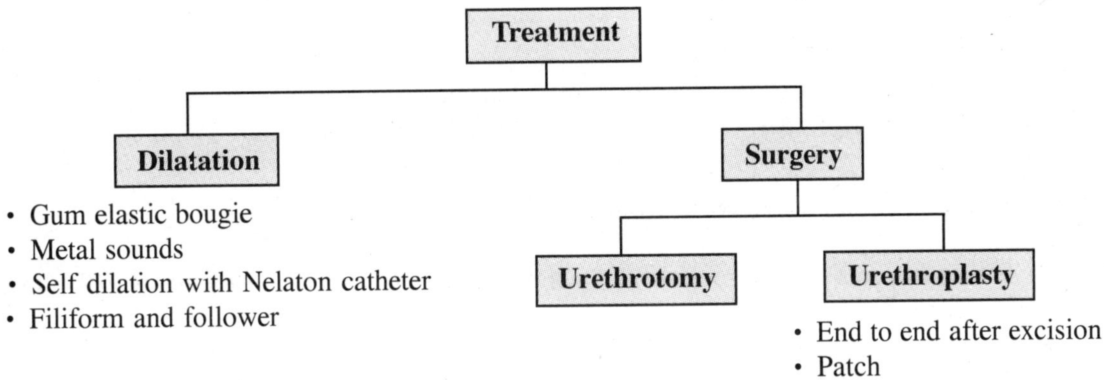

SAQ 7 What are different neoplasms of urethra?

(i) Polyp
(ii) Genital warts
(iii) Mutifocal transitional cell cancers, squamous carcinoma
(iv) Angioma of urethra

SAQ 8 What is fracture penis?

It occurs due to errect penis is bent downwards, treated by incision and drainage of clot and suture of the tunica corpus cavernosum.

SAQ 9 What is paraphimosis?

Paraphimosis occurs when the tight foreskin is difficult to return, causing obstruction of venous and lymphatic return of the glan's distal to foreskin.

SAQ 10 What is balanoposthitis?

Inflammation of glans = Balantitis
Inflammation of prepuce = Posthitis

SAQ 11 What is chordae?

Fixed bowing of penis, may be due to chronic urethritis or hypospadius. Treatment is surgical repair.

SAQ 12 What is priapism?

It is painful errection of penis as in:

- Sickle cell disease
- Injection of papaverine
- Leukemia
- Spinal cord disease

SAQ 13 What is erythroplasia of Querat?

Paget's disease of penis or erythroplasia of Querat is persistant rawness of the glans (balantitis), followed by cancer.

SAQ 14 What is Buschke-Lowenstein tumour of penis?

Histologically verrucous carcinoma of penis locally invasive and destructive. Treated surgically.

34 Testis and Scrotum

SAQ 1 What are the layers of scrotum?

It has following layers from outside inwards:

(i) Skin
(ii) Dartos
(iii) External aponeurosis
(iv) Creamester
(v) Internal aponeurosis
(vi) Tunica vaginalis.

SAQ 2 How the testis develops?

It develops from genital fold lying medial to wolffian duct in lumbar region. Mesonephros disappear, only few of its tubule remains as vas efferentia. Wolffian duct becomes epididymis and vas deferens. Gubernaculum testis brings it down to scrotum which provides optimum temperature for spermatogenesis.

SAQ 3 What are the complications of undescended testis?

(i) Sterility
(ii) Malignancy
(iii) Pain due to trauma
(iv) Torsion
(v) Epididymo-orchitis
(vi) Indirect inguinal hernia

SAQ 4 What are probable sites of undescended testis?

The gubernaculum testis may bring down the testis to any of its attachment sites. It may be:

- Intraabdominal
- At inguinal canal
- Superficial inguinal pouch.

SAQ 5 How to treat undescended testis?

(i) Orchidopexy
(ii) HCG hormone if hypogonadism
(iii) Orchidectomy if other testis is normal

LAQ 6 What are the predisposing causes of torsion of spermatic cord (torsion of testis)? How it presents?

Causes of torsion of testis

(i) Inversion of testis
(ii) High investment of the tunica vaginalis
(iii) Separation of epididymis from body of testis

Presentation

- Pain
- Vomiting
- Thickened tender cord
- Doppler ultrasound scan will show absence of blood supply to the affected testis.

SAQ 7 What is varicocele?

It is the varicose dilatation of the veins draining testis, mostly (95%) in left testis. It may cause primary infertility.

Ligation of testicular vein above inguinal ligament where pampiniform plexus coalesced into one or two vessels are done, if producing symptoms.

SAQ 8 What is hydrocele?

It is abnormal collection of serous fluid in processus vaginalis (generally tunica vaginalis) due to:

(i) Excess production
(ii) Defective absorption of fluid
(iii) Connection of hernia with peritoneal sac
(iv) Lymphatic drainage of scrotum is obstructed

SAQ 9 Mention important diagnostic tests for hydrocele.

- Get above the swelling
- Scrotal swelling
- Translucency

SAQ 10 What are the complications of hydrocele?

The complications of hydrocele are:

- Rupture
- Calcification
- Infection
- Haemorrhage Malignancy (rare)

SAQ 11 What are the different operations for hydrocele?

(i) Lord's operation
(ii) Jabaulay's operation
(iii) Filarial hydrocele is treated by rest, aspiration and excision of sac
(iv) Haematocele is drained

SAQ 12 Name the different cysts connected to epididymis.

(i) Epididymal cyst
(ii) Cyst in the appendages of testicle
(iii) Spermatocele

LAQ 13 Write short notes on epididymo-orchitis.

Inflammation of epididymis is epididymitis and that of testis is orchitis

Epididymo-orchitis

Acute	Chronic
Reaches via vas from primary infection of urethra, prostate, seminal vesicle, STD of (chlamydia, gonococcal).	Tuberculosis
Clinical features of prostitis: Ache in groin fever, scrotum (is red, shiny oedematous, may be with pus discharging)	Clinical feature: Pain on lower pole of epididymis which aches a little, secondary hydrocele, seminal vesicles indurated, renal Tb may be there
Treatment: Antibiotics after C/S if possible doxycycline, plenty of fluid, pain releif. Testis may atrophy	ATD; Epididectomy or orchidectomy if there is no resolution after 2–6 weeks of conservative treatment

SAQ 14 What are the different types of testicular tumours?

- Seminoma
- Seminoma and teratoma
- Teratoma
- Interstitial tumour, lymphoma

LAQ 15 Write short note on seminoma.

Macroscopically: Smooth and firm, cut surface is pinkish, cream colour, with fibrous septa giving lobulated appearance with areas of necrosis.

Microscopically: Oval cells, rounded nuclei and nucleoli, clear cytoplasm. Cells arranged in sheets with fibrous stroma.

Origin: Seminiferous tubule.

Spread: Mostly lymphatics.

LAQ 16 Write short note on teratoma.

Origin: Rete testis.
Size: Peanut to coconut, covered by tunica albuginea.

It may be classified as following:

(i) Teratoma differentiated
(ii) Malignant teratoma intermediate (MTI)
(iii) Malignant teratoma anaplastic (MTA)
(iv) Malignant teratoma trophoblastic (MTT)

SAQ 17 Name the different interstitial cell tumours.

It may arise from Leydig (masculinising) or from Sertoli cell tumour (feminising).

LAQ 18 How a testicular tumour presents?

Lump in testes (enlarged, smooth, firm); pain, loss of testicular sensation, secondary hydrocele thickening of spermatic cord, creamasteric hypertrophy; enlarged testicular vessels; PR: prostate normal; secondary retroperitoneal deposit and other signs of malignant deposits.

(i) Stage1: Only testicular lesion
(ii) Stage2: Involves lymph node below diaphragm
(iii) Stage3: Involves lymph nodes above diaphragm
(iv) Stage4: Pulmonary and hepatic spread.

SAQ 19 Name the different types of treatment for testicular tumour.

(i) Surgery (scrotal exploration with orchidectomy)
(ii) Radiotherapy: (seminomas are radiosensitive; teratomas are less sensitive)
(iii) Chemotherapy (cisplatin; methotrexate; bleomycin for teratoma and retroperitoneal spread).

SAQ 20 Name a testicular tumour of children.

It generally occurs before three years and is anaplastic teratoma.

SAQ 21 What are the causes of infertility in male?

(i) Failure in act of performance of coitus
(ii) Failure in conductance of sperms
(iii) Failure in formation of sperms (azoospermia)

LAQ 22 What is Fournier's gangrene?

Idiopathic scrotal gangrene or Fournier's gangrene is vascular disease of infective origin characterised by sudden scrotal inflammation with gangrene causing rupture of scrotal contents. *Strepto, Staph, Cl.welchii, E.coli,* etc. cause obliterative arteritis.

Presentation: Pain in scrotum, fever, prostration, pallor, cellulites

Treatment: Excision of necrotic skin and antibiotics (gentamicin and chephalosporin)

Prognosis: Patient may die even after active treatment.

35 Jaw, Lips, Palate, Face and Mouth

SAQ 1 What is epulis?

Epulis literally mean situated on the gum. Pathologically, it means outgrowth from alveolar process.

LAQ 2 Classify jaw tumours.

- **Epulis**
  - **Benign**
    - Fibroid
    - Giant cells
    - Melanotic
  - **Malignant**
    - Fibrosarcomatous
    - Epithelioma
- **Odontomes**
  - **From enamel**
    - Dental cyst
    - Adamantinoma
  - **Odontomes of dental sac**
    - Dentigerous cyst
    - Fibrous odontome
    - Cementome
    - Compound follicular odontoma
  - **Odontome from dental papilla**
    - Radicular odontoma
  - **Odontome from whole tooth**
    - Composite odontoma
- **Benign tumours of jaw bone**
  - Ossifying fibroma
  - Fibrous osteoma
  - Fibrous dysplasia
  - Osteoma
  - Paget's disease
  - Osteoclastoma
  - Solitary cyst
  - Myxoma
  - Hyperparathyroidism
- **Malignant tumours of jaw bones**
  - Carcinoma
  - Sarcoma (osteogenic)
  - Lymphoepithelioma
  - Burkitt's lymphoma

LAQ 3 Mention in brief the development of palate and lips.

Stomodeal depression occurs on cephalic end of foetus around which there are five elevated process develop, called frotonasal process; two maxillary laterally and two mandibular processes at lower end.

Two olfactory pits develop in frontonasal process and divide the fontonasal process into one median nasal process and two lateral nasal processes. Lateral nasal process fuses maxillary process. Median nasal process produces philtrum and upper lip and lateral parts of upper lip are produced. Shelves like projection from median nasal process called premaxilla and from two maxillary processes on either side called palatine process fuse to produce palate.

SAQ 4 How the cleft lip and palate are classified?

Recently, it is classified on LAHS where L = lip; A = alveolus; H = hard palate; S = soft palate. Capital letter means complete cleft and small letter means incomplete cleft. LAHSHAL is complete bilateral cleft.

SAQ 5 When to operate cleft lip? What are the operations called?

Preferably within 48 hours, because of maternal antibodies or at 6 months or 2 pound of weight when baby can stand anaesthesia.

Late operations are not satisfactory. Operation is called Mirault-Blair operation where misplaced tissues are repaired to bring normal appearance of lip; nose.

SAQ 6 What are different types of cleft palate?

It may be tripartite Y; bipartite Y; intermaxillary complete or incomplete. Complicated with cleft lip or uncomplicated.

SAQ 7 What difficulties may arise out of cleft palate?

(i) Inability to suck (ii) Regurgitation of food (iii) Dental crippling

SAQ 8 What are the different operations of cleft palate and what is the ideal age of operation?

Different operations are:

(i) Two flap operation (Langenbeck's operation)
(ii) Four flap (Wardill's operation)

British surgeons prefer when child gets 14 lb weight after 6 months, but before 18 months before childs starts speaking.

SAQ 9 What secondary managements are required after cleft lip management?

These are:

(i) Hearing (conductive; sensorineuronal)
(ii) Speech (velopharyngeal incompetence; articulation problem)
(iii) Dental developmental problem
(iv) Facial growth problem, etc. has to be managed.

SAQ 10 What are the different causes of defective tooth structure?

(i) Amelogenesis imperfecta
(ii) Dentinogenous imperfecta
(iii) Trauma
(iv) Measles
(v) Rickets
(vi) Fluoride
(vii) Tetracycline

36 Salivary Gland

SAQ 1 What is pes anserinus?

The VII CN after coming out of stytomastoid foramen, first devides into temporofacial and cervico-facial division and then into varing member of branches interconnected like goose feet (pes anserinus).

SAQ 2 What are the parts of parotid gland?

Superficial part, deep part, accessory parotids and parotid duct (Stensen's duct) which after receiving interlobular ducts opens into the mouth via small papilla opposite second upper molar tooth inside the cheek.

SAQ 3 What are the parts of submandibular glands?

Superficial, deep parts and Wharton's duct.

SAQ 4 What is sialography?

Here radiograph is taken after introducing radio-opaque liquid (sodium diatrizoate) or lipiodal in the duct system of parotid or submandibular gland to visualize outline of lumen of the duct, salivary neoplasm, fistulae, neoplasm, etc.

SAQ 5 What are the causes of acute parotitis?

- Viral: (Mumps coxsackie virus, etc.)
- During debilitating infection (typhoid, cholera)
- Sjögren's syndrome (by autoantibodies)
- Tuberculosis
- Following major surgery
- After radiotherapy

SAQ 6 What is the cause of acute suppurative sialoadenitis of submandibular gland?

It occurs as a consequence of obstruction of Wharton's gland.

LAQ 7 What are the different neoplasms of salivary glands?

- **Epithelial tumours**
  - **Adenoma**
    - Pleomorphic mixed
    - Monomorphic
      - Adenolymphoma
      - Oxyphilic
      - Others
  - **Mucoepidermoid**

- **Non-epithelial tumour**
  - **Acinic cell tumour**
  - **Carcinoma**
    - Adenoid cystic carcinoma
    - Adenocarcinoma
    - Epidermoid carcinoma
    - Undifferentiated carcinoma
    - Ca of pleomorphic adenoma

SAQ 8 Write short note on pleomorphic adenoma of salivary gland.

Here epithelial cells proliferate and some arrange like ducts, and myoepithelial cells proliferate like sheets. Mucoid materials are produced to produce myxomatous appearance like cartilage. May be cystic, presents as firm elastic, lobulated. May show signs of malignancy after 10–30 years.

SAQ 9 What is Frey syndrome or auriculotemporal syndrome?

Here there flushing and sweating of skin innervated by auriculotemporal nerve occurs after surgery of that region or TM joint or accidentally or due to birth trauma.

SAQ 10 What is Sjögren's syndrome?

Rheumatoid arthritis + Dry eyes + Dry mouth. Maybe SLE or scleroderma.

LAQ 11 What is Mikulicz disease?

(i) Symmetrical enlargement of all salivary glands
(ii) Narrowing of palpebral fissures due to enlargement of lacrimal glands
(iii) Parchment dryness of the mouth.

Treated by obliterating lacrimal punctum by diathermy and using artificial tear methyl cellulose, oral hygine, 1% chlorhexidine gluconate), steroids and immunosuppressants.

SAQ 12 What is sialosis?

This is enlargement of salivary glands for metabolic reasons (diabetes; acromegaly patient on bizarre diet and overweight).

37 Neck

SAQ 1 What is branchial cyst? How it presents and treated?

Generally arises from 2nd branchial cleft which is a vestigial organ. Lined by squamous epithelium containing clear or toothpaste like fluid. Appear after 20 years protruding beneath the anterior border of sternomastoid as fluctuating and transilluminating swelling, containing cholesterol crystals. It may be infected.

Treated by excision.

SAQ 2 What is branchial fistula?

These are persistant 2nd branchial cleft, the occluding membrane of which is broken down. The external orifice of this fistula is near the lower end of anterior broder of sternomastoid muscle. It is lined columnar ciliated epithelium, discharge mucus and prone to recurrent infection. It should be excised if producing troublesome infection.

LAQ 3 Write notes on cavernous lymphangioma (cystic hygroma).

Primitive lymph sac develops in mesoblast in the region of neck. Sequestration of jugular lymph sac produces cystic hygroma generally occurs at neck, axilla.

Presentation: Presents from birth, may cause obstructed labour. Found generally in neck as intercommunicating fluid containing compartments containing fluids. Size increases on coughing, crying. The cysts are fluctuating, transilluminant.

Complication: (i) Infection and (ii) respiratory obstruction

Treatment: Excision. In order to check growth of cyst and making it fibrous 3–6 injections of boiling water is given into the cyst at weekly intervals.

Complications: (i) Recurrence, (ii) leakage of lymph, (iii) surgical anaesthetic risks.

LAQ 4 What is cervical rib? What are their varieties? How they present clinically?

The remnant of costal element of cervical ribs are called cervical ribs.

Types: (i) **Complete**

(ii) **Incomplete**
- Free end expands as bony
- Ending in tapering point
- Ending in fibrous band

Cervical rib—clinical presentation

Local symptoms

Lump in lower neck

Vascular symptoms

- Pain
- Numbness
- Temperature and colour changes
- Systolic bruit in subclavian artery

Nerve symptoms

- Pain
- Tingling and wasting of thener and hypothener muscles

Treatment: (i) Sling and exercise

(ii) Sclerotomy

(iii) Removal of cervical rib from periosteum to avoid regenerate

SAQ 5 What are the complications of the throat injury?

- Haemorrhage
- Pneumonia
- Emphysema
- Embolism
- Fistula (of larynx or trachea, oesophagus)
- Dysphonia or aphonia
- Infection

SAQ 6 What is potato tumour or carotid body tumour?

Histologically, it is non-chromaffin preganglioma (chemodectoma).

Occurs in carotid body (mostly of chemoreceptor system). May remain localized for years and then metastasizes locally and less likely distantly.

LAQ 7 What are the causes of cervical lymphadenopathy?

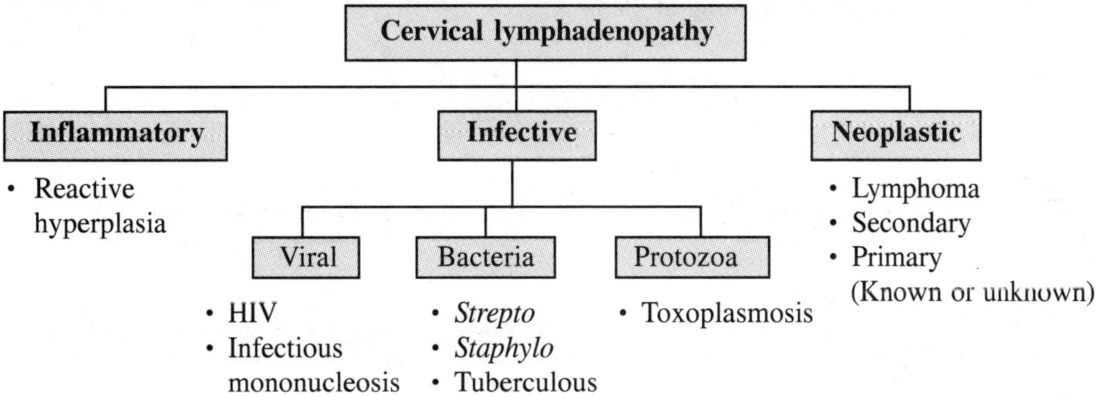

SAQ 8 What are the different types of neck dissection?

The different types of neck dissection are following:

(i) **Classical radical neck dissection**
(ii) **Modified radical neck dissection** (accessory nerve, sternomastoid, internal jugular vein are preserved)
(iii) **Selective neck dissection**

SAQ 9 What is torticolis?

In torticolis or wry neck, the head is bent to one side and cheek to the other side. It may be:

(i) Congenital
(ii) Traumatic
(iii) Rheumatic
(iv) Reflex
(v) Spasmodic
(vi) Compensatory
(vii) Pott's disease

In long-standing cases, there may be atrophy of muscle. Measurement of outer canthus to angle of mouth is smaller, eyebrows are less arched.

SAQ 10 What are the different tumours of the neck?

(i) Chemodectoma (cortid body tumours)
(ii) Vagal body tumours
(iii) Peripheral nerve tumours (neurofibroma)
(iv) Secondary carcinoma

SAQ 11 What are the causes of swelling of the neck?

Following are the causes of swelling of the neck:

Neck swellings

- **Superficial to deep fascia**
  - Sebaceous cyst
  - Lipoma
  - Carbuncle
  - Neurofibroma
- **Deep-to-deep fascia**
  - **Lateral swellings**
    - Lymph node
    - Thyroid
    - Branchial cyst
    - Sternomastoid tumour
    - Cervical rib
    - Cystic hygroma
    - Aneurysm
    - Carotid body tumour
    - Salivary gland
    - Actinomycosis
    - Muscle
    - Tumour
    - Clavicular tumour
  - **Midline swellings**
    - Thyroglossal cyst
    - Pharyngeal pouch
    - Subhyoid bursa
    - Laryngocele
    - Plunging ranula
    - Ca larynx or trachea
    - Perichondritis of thyroid cartilage.

38 Chest

SAQ. 1 Describe the peculiarities of right and left lungs and right and left bronchus.

Left lung is devided by oblique fissure into upper lobes whereas right lungs upper lobe is further divided to middle lobe.

Right main bronchus is straight and shorter, therefore foreign body is likely to enter this lobe.

SAQ 2 Which patients are fit for lung resection?

Patient with $FEV_1 > 1.5$ litres are fit for lung resection.

SAQ 3 What is stove in the chest and flail chest?

Fracture of several consecutive ribs produces stove in the chest and when it looses the support, it is called flail chest.

LAQ. 4 What is the mechanism of paradoxical respiration and mediastinal flutter?

A large opening of chest wall causes shrinking of affected side during inspiration and air in pleural space pushes the mediastinum towards healthy side and areation of unaffected lung is also impaired. During expiration, air passes from good lung towards collapsed lung this side to side movement is called mediastinal flutter and respiration is paradoxical respiration.

SAQ 5 What is pneumothorax?

It is air outside lungs within pleural space. It may be spontaneous (primary and secondary); tension. In tension pneumothorax, there is positive pressure within hemithorax leading to:

(i) Collapsed lung
(ii) Flattened diaphragm
(iii) Mediastinal distortion
(iv) Impaired venous return to heart

SAQ 6 What is surgical emphysema?

It is air in the soft tissue due to communication of air containing viscus to soft tissue.

Important causes are: (i) Rupture oesophagus, surgical, mediastinal surgical emphysema may occur in asthma in ventilator, barotrauma patient.

LAQ 7 What are the different methods of treatment for pneumothorax?

(i) If the patient is comfortable watch the patient and monitor PO_2
(ii) Drain immediately breathless hypoxic patient
(iii) Pleurectomy and pleurodesis
(iv) **V**ideo-**a**ssisted **t**horacoscopic **s**urgery (**VATS**)

VATS objectives

- To deal leaks of lungs
- To search belbs and treat it.
- Pleural adhesion
  - Pleurectomy
  - Chemical pleurodesis
  - Pleural abrasion

LAQ 8 Mention the important uses of bronchoscopy.

INDICATIONS OF BRONCHOSCOPE

Diagnostic
- To confirm Ca bronchus, vocal cord palsy, etc.
- Tissue biopsy, septum

Preoperative
- In haemoptysis
- Before oesophageal and lung resection

Therapeutic
- Removal of foreign bodies or secretion, stent placing

LAQ 9 What is empyema? What are the important causes of it?

It is thick pus or coagulum with thick cortex of fibrin over the lung. It has generally three phases
• Exudative phase • Fibrinopurulant phase • Organising phase

Etiologies

From outside
- Haemothorax
- Penetrating wound
- Repeated aspiration

Chest wall
- Osteomyelitis
- Abscess
- Ca lung
- Bronchectasis
- Actinomycosis

Form lung
- Pneumonia
- Lung abscess

Oesophagus
- Ca
- Rupture

Below diaphragm
- Subphrenic abscess

SAQ 10 What are the indications of surgery in tuberculosis?

Tuberculosis per se is treated by medicine, may require surgery, if there is suspicion of:
- Chronic abscess resistant to chemotherapy
- With severe haemoptysis
- With aspergilloma of tuberculous cavity.

SAQ 11 Name some medical conditions in chest which may require surgery.

(i) Bronchiectasis, (ii) lung abscess, (iii) tuberculosis

LAQ 12 What are the important indications of lung transplantations?

It is indicated for end stage lung parenchymal or pulmonary vascular diseases, viz. cystic fibrosis, pulmonary fibrosis, obstructive airway disease in young, etc. The different types are: One donor lung; two donor lung or heart lung block.

Apart from precautions of organ matching, cytomegalovirus status is important to prevent CMV pneumonitis.

SAQ 13 What are the complications of fracture ribs?

- Shock
- Surgical emphysema
- Wet lung
- Subdiaphragmatic injury (liver; spleen; kidney; gut; hernia)
- Pneumo- or haemothorax
- Stove and flail in chest
- Contusion or laceration of lung

LAQ 14 Describe the following (i) Cervical ribs, (ii) pectus excavatum, (iii) pectus carinatum.

Cervical ribs: A fibrous band from 7th cervical vertibra and inserting 1st thoracic rib. May be asymptomatic or with different neurovascular symptoms.

Pectus excavatum: Here sternum is depressed with dish-shaped deformity

Pectus carinatum: Sternum is elevated above ribs. Surgery required for cosmetic regions.

39 Cardiac Surgery

SAQ 1 Mention the important complications of cardiopulmonary bypass.

- Bleeding
- Ischaemia
- Cholecystitis
- Pulmonary and vascular injury
- Infection
- Temponade
- Pancreatitis
- Neurological and systemic organ dysfunctions.
- Pericarditis
- Myocardial depression
- Postcardiotomy syndrome

LAQ 2 What are the different methods of diagnosing ischaemic cardiac disease?

Diagnostic methods of ishaemic heart disease

Non-invasive methods

- Resting ECG
- Cardiac isoenzymes and troponin (for actue syndrome)
- Exercise tolerance testing
- Echocardiogram
- Radionucleotide studies
- PET

Invasive methods

- Coronary angiogram

SAQ 3 What are the different modes of treatment of myocardial infarction?

The different modes of treatment of myocardial infarction are:

- Thrombolysis
- PTCA
- CABG

SAQ 4 What are the contraindications of CABG?

- Diffusely diseased arteries
- AMI over 6 hours
- Patient with heart failure
- Moribund patient with lengthy resuscitation

SAQ 5 What is Euroscore?

This is risk stratification with scoring system done for cardiac surgery (**E**uropean **S**ystem for **C**ardiac **O**perative **R**isk **E**valuation). Other method is Parsonnet; Ontario scoring system.

SAQ 6 Which veins or arteries are selected for conduit?

(i) Long saphenous vein
(ii) Short saphenous vein
(iii) Cephalic vein
(iv) Left internal mammary artery
(v) Bilateral internal artery
(vi) Radial artery

SAQ 7 What is Allen's test?

It is a test to assess in whom radial artery harvest has been planned. Patient makes a tight fist and surgeon compresses ulnar artery. Patient fist and ulnar artery is released to see speed of recovery, if colour comes in 5–7 seconds, ulnar collaterals are patent.

SAQ 8 What postoperative complications may arise of CABG operation?

(i) Bleeding
(ii) Arrhythmia
(iii) Poor cardiac output
(iv) Wound infection
(v) Neurological deficit.

SAQ 9 What are different types of prosthetic valves?

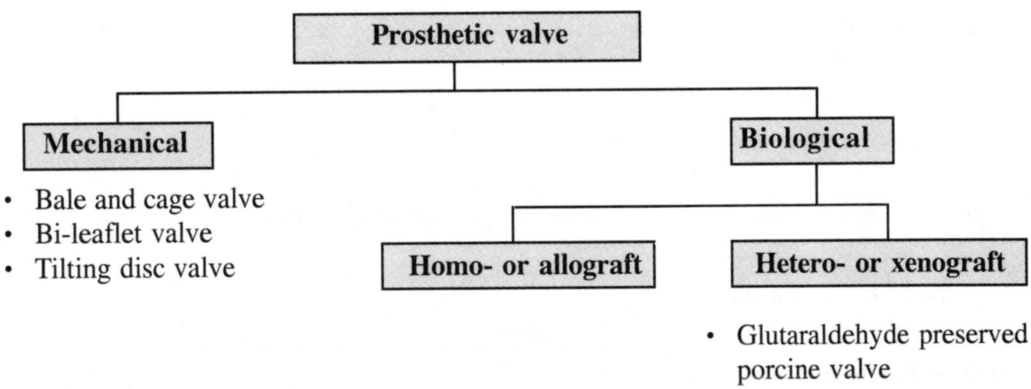

SAQ 10 What complications may arise out of prosthetic valve and how they are managed?

- Structural valve failure
- Thrombosis
- Leak
- Endocarditis

Managed with:

- Antibiotics
- Antithrombotic

SAQ 11 Classify heart failure functionally (New York Heart Association).

Class I	Class II	Class III	Class IV
Asymptomatic without physical limitation	Mild symptoms on activities of daily living	Difficulties in doing activities of daily	Short of breath to do simple activities

SAQ 12 What are the indications of operation in mitral stenosis?

(i) Severe symptoms III and IV
(ii) Mitral stenosis with valve area 1.5 cm^2
(iii) With emboli

SAQ 13 What are the different types of operations for mitral valve?

These are:

(i) Closed mitral valvotomy
(ii) Open mitral valvotomy
(iii) Mitral valve repair (prosthetic ring annuloplasty; quadrangular resection of posterior leaflet sliding plasty, chordal shortening, chordal transposition)
(iv) Mitral valve replacement

SAQ 14 What are the indications of surgery in aortic stenosis?

(i) Systemic hypotension
(ii) Arterial vasodilatation

→ Producing myocardial ischaemia

SAQ 15 What are the indications of surgery in aortic incompetence?

- Cardiac failure III and IV of NYHA
- End diastolic and systolic dimension > 70 and 50 mm respectively
- End diastolic and systolic pressure 70 and 50 mm Hg, respectively

SAQ 16 What are the cardiac lesions of Fallot's tetralogy?

- Over riding of arota
- VSD
- Pulmonary stenosis
- RVH

SAQ 17 What are the different operations for Fallot's operation?

- Left subclavian and pulmonary artery shunt (Blalock-Taussig operation)
- Aorta and right pulmonary artery shunt of Waterstone
- Descending arota and left pulmonary artery shunt of Pott.

SAQ 18 What are the contraindications of cardiac transplantation?

Absolute:

(i) Other life-threatening disease like malignancy, HIV infection
(ii) Irreversible pulmonary hypertension

Relative: • Age more than 60 • Poor creatinine clearance • Psychiatric illness • Drug abuse

SAQ 19 Mention the criteria of selection of cardiac donar.

- Male with 45 years and female with 50 years
- ABO matching
- HB or bacterial infection
- Weight should be 25% of receipient
- Not on inotropic or with HIV
- Without coronary artery disease.

SAQ 20 What postoperative complications may arise of mitral valvotomy?

Closed or open mitral valvotomy may produce following complications:

(i) Embolism (systemic or pulmonary)
(ii) Suppurative bronchitis
(iii) Cardiac failure
(iv) Rhythm disorders

SAQ 21 What are the indications of surgery for ASD?

(i) Osteum secundum ASD not closing spontaneously
(ii) Osteum primum ASD with left to right shunt 1.5:1

SAQ 22 What are the indications of surgery for VSD?

(i) Large defect
(ii) Fails to manage medically
(iii) Left to right shunt 2:1 with increasing pulmonary vascular resistance
(iv) VSD with complications like AI, infundibular stenosis, IE, pleurisy, pneumonia.

SAQ 23 What are the causes of acute temponade?

- Trauma
- Dissecting aneurysm
- Iatrogenic

SAQ 24 What is aneurysm?

Aneurysm is blood space or sac formed by widening of the lumen of the artery due to weakness of the arterial wall (congenital; traumatic, pathological)

Classical:

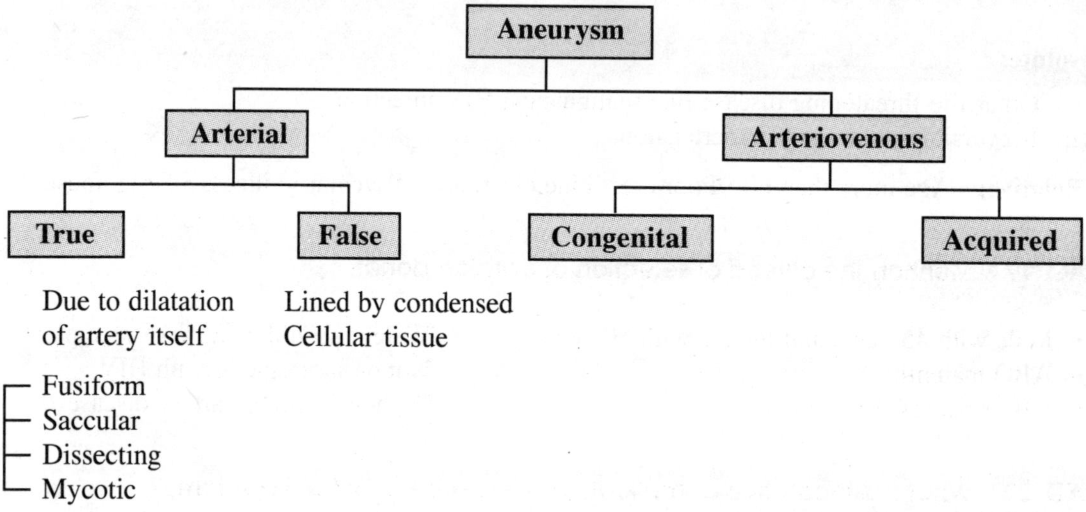

40 Breast

SAQ 1 Describe the anatomical position of the breast.

Protuberant part of the human breast lies over 2–6 ribs from lateral border of sternum to anterior axillary line.

SAQ 2 What is surgical importance of axillary tail?

It may be normally palpable or in premenstruation or lactation and may be mistaken for lymph node, lipoma or breast lump.

LAQ 3 Mention the lymphatic drainage of the breast.

Eighty-five per cent of the lymphatic drainage of breast drain into axillary and internal mammary lymph nodes as following:

1. Lateral along axillary vein
2. Central embedded in the fats of centre of the axilla
3. Anterior along lateral thoracic vessels
4. Posterior along subscapular vessels
5. Interpectoral lying between pectoris major and minor

LAQ 4 Mention the important investigations of breasts.

(i) Mammography safe investigation, sensitivity increases with age because breast becomes less dense. Breast is exposed to low voltage and high amperage X-ray and the breast is placed on ultrasensitive films.

(ii) USG: Helps distinguishing cyst from solid and in dense breast of youngs

(iii) MRI

(iv) Needle biopsy (FNAC) and cytology. Obtained by using 21 or 23 G needle with 10 ml syringe

(v) Galactography

(vi) Thermography

SAQ 5 What is triple assessment?

Diagnosis of suspicious breast cancer made on:
(i) Clinical assessment
(ii) Radiology and
(iii) Cytology or histology is called triple assessment

SAQ 6 Wrtie short note on retracted nipple.

Maybe before puberty, if occurs after puberty is called simple nipple inversion (etiology unknown), may cause difficulties in breastfeeding or infection. Recent retraction signifies significant pathology.

Treated by:
(i) Mechanical suction or by (ii) Surgical correction. It may resolve spontaneously also.

SAQ 7 Name the common congenital anomalies of the breast.

1. Amazia (absence of one or both breast)
2. Polymazia (accessory breast)
3. Athelia (absence of nipple)
4. Polythelia (accessory nipple)
5. Congenital retracted nipple

LAQ 8 Write short note on discharge from nipple.

Note the following

1. Nature, quantity and duration of discharge
   - Blood stained (duct papilloma or carcinoma)
   - Serous (fibroadenosis, physiological)
   - Greenish (fibroadenosis, duct ectasia)
   - Blackish (papilloma or carcinoma of duct)
   - Milk (Galactocele or duct ectasia) hypothyroid
   - Creamy (duct ectasia)
   - Purulent (mamillary fistula, infection)
2. Whether associated with lump?
3. How started? Whether with pain?
4. Whether localized to one or more ducts?

SAQ 9 What is Mondor's disease?

Thrombophlebitis of superficial veins of breast of anterior chest wall or in arm is called Mondor's disease.

By restriction of arm movement, it resolves spontaneously generally, without recurrence complications or deformity.

It should be differentiated from occult carcinoma of breast.

SAQ 10 What is Paget's disease of the breast?

It is a persistant eczema-like condition of nipple appears after 50 years and does not respond to treatment, slowly progresses peripherally to produce carcinoma of breast. It is slowly growing duct carcinoma infiltrating epithelium of nipple.

SAQ 11 What are the important differential diagnois of breast pain and how to treat it?

- Abscess
- Fibroadenosis
- Carcinoma
- Chondritis

If the pain is not due to cancer, reassure the patient, suggest her firm bra at day and soft bra at night. Oil of evening primrose, danazol 100 mg to start with and increase up to 100 mg TDS. Other drugs are bromocriptine; tamoxifen or LHRH.

LAQ 12 What is cystosarcoma phylloides of breast?

This is soft fibroadenoma, due to growth, degeneration and cyst formation, also called serocystic disease of Brodie which appear like leaves (phylloides) side by side therefore also called **cystosarcoma of phylloides**. When it fungates through skin called **cystosarcoma fungoides.**

There is no pain, fixicity, involvement of lymph node. Some have malignant potential and some have high mitotic index. May metastasise by bloodstream.

Treated by enucleation in young. Recurrent or massive or malignant type require mastectomy.

LAQ 13 What are the etiological factors of Ca breast?

- Geographical factors (more in western world)
- Less common in male
- Less below 20 years
- Common with family history of Ca breast
- Common in alcoholics with diet low in phytoestrogens
- Common in nulliparous
- Postmenopausal woman
- Role of OCP is doubtful; milk factors

SAQ 14 What is peau d'orange?

It is cutaneous lymphatic oedema of infiltrated skin is tethered by sweat ducts which cannot swell, so look like orange skin.

SAQ 15 What is cancer en cuirasse?

Here due to infiltration of the skin of the chest by Ca breast, looks like a coat, may be associated with swollen arm.

SAQ 16 What is lymphangiosarcoma?

Lymphangiosarcoma may occur as lymphoedema in a casé of Ca breast following its treatment, presents as multiple subcutaneous nodule in the upper limb. May responds to cytotoxic drugs or radiation. Interscapulothoracic amputation is indicated at times.

SAQ 17 How the breast Ca is staged?

They are staged according to Manchester system and international union against cancer (tumour; nodes; metastases, i.e. TNM system).

SAQ 18 Mention the prognosis of breast cancer.

It depends upon its chronological age, invasive potential, histological grade, S phase fraction, tymidine labelling index, growth factor analysis, oncogenes product, tumour size and lymph node status. Though some large tumours are local and many small tumours are incurable.

SAQ 19 What is Patey's mastectomy?

Here breast and associated structures (large portion of skin over tumour, nipple, fat fascia, and lymph nodes of the axilla) are excised.

SAQ 20 What is QUART?

Quadranectomy, **A**xillary dissection + **R**adiotherapy helps preventing recurrence, though overall outcome is unchanged.

SAQ 21 What is sentinel lymph node biopsy?

Sentinel lymph nodes are localized by injecting radio-isotope or patent blue dye arround the tumour and the draining nodes are biopsied. If the lymph node is biophysically negative, then axillary dissection can be avoided.

LAQ 22 What are the other modes of treatment of breast cancer apart from surgery?

(i) Adjuvant therapy with hormones (tamoxifen, LHRH agonist)
(ii) Chemotherapy with cyclophosphamide, methotrexate and 5FU
(iii) Breast reconstruction
(iv) Immunotherapy
(v) Irradiation
(vi) Hypophysectomy, adrenalectomy, oophorectomy

LAQ 23 What are the causes of gynaecomastia?

In gynaecomastia, male breasts look like female (uni- or bilaterally)

Causes I—**Idiopathic** (crossed puberty)

II—**Secondary**: Oestrogen therapy for Ca prostate patient, testicular tumour (chorioepithelioma), mumps, castration, adrenal and pituitary tumours, Klinefelter's syndrome, cirrhosis, leprosy, Ca of bronchus.

Treated by mastectomy (breast tissue is scrapped from inside).

SAQ 24 What is traumatic fat necrosis of breast?

Here aseptic saponification of neutral fat of breast occurs due to trauma (known or unknown)

LAQ 25 Mention the different types of cyst of breast.

Breast cysts

- **Due to mammary dysplasia**
  - Single (blue domed cyst of blood good)
  - Multiple
- **Retention cyst**
  - Galactocele
- **Tumour cyst**
  - **Benign**
    - Cystosarcoma phylloides
    - Papillary cystadenoma
  - **Malignant**
    - Colloid degeneration
    - Intracyst
- **Miscellaneous**
  - Blood cyst
  - Lymphatic cyst
  - Dermoid cyst
  - Hydatid cyst

LAQ 26 Mention the different benign neoplasms of the breasts.

Benign neoplasms of breast

- **Epithelial origin**
  - Duct papilloma
  - Pure adenoma
- **Connective tissue origin**
  - Neurofibroma
  - Lipoma
- **Mixed origin**
  - Fibroadenoma (intracanalicular, pericanalicular)
  - Papillary cystadenoma

LAQ 27 What are the different clinical types of carcinoma breast?

- Mastitis carcinomatosis
- Scirrhous carcinoma
- Duct carcinoma
- Paget's disease of nipple
- Pseudolipoma
- Medullary carcinoma
- Atropic scirrhous carcinoma
- Intracystic papilliferous carcinoma
- Sarcoma

41 Diseases of Bones and Joints

SAQ 1 What are the points to be observed in locomotor system?

In locomotor system's examination: (GALS)

(i) Gait, (ii) arms, (iii) legs, (iv) spines to be examined thoroughly.

SAQ 2 What is skeletal dysplasias?

Skeletal dysplasias are monogenic disease of bones and cartilage matrix, viz. osteogenesis imperfecta, osteopetrosis, hypophosphatasia.

In chondrodysplasia, primarily cartilage development is defective.

SAQ 3 What do you mean osteogenesis imperfecta?

In this skeletal dysplasia condition, there is abnormalities of type I collagen leading to qualitative and quantitative deficiency of bony matrix with fracture risks, stunting of growth, defective dentinogenesis, hearing loss, blue sclera, hypermobile joint, skin laxity, scaring reminiscent of skin.

It is treated by bisphosphonates and orthopaedic surgery for fractures.

SAQ 4 What is osteopetrosis or marble bone disease?

Osteopetrosis is genetically recessively transmitted, with increased bone density and fragility.

There is mutation in osteoclast specific proton pump or mutation in carbonic anhydrase gene. Bone marrow failure and splenic enlargement is common.

SAQ 5 What is hypophosphatasia?

In hypophosphatasia, variable deficiency of bone mineralization occurs due to mutation of alkaline phosphatase gene. May cause fracture in utero, cranial synostosis, teeth abnormalities, low alkaline phosphatase and phosphoethanolaminuria.

SAQ 6 What is chondrodysplasia?

These are defects of cartilage and endochondrial ossification, viz. achondroplasia, spondyloepiphyseal dysplasia, multiple epiphyseal dysplasia, metaphyseal dysplasia, craniofrontal dysplasia, diastrophic dysplasia.

LAQ 7 What is Marfan's syndrome? Mention the indications of surgery in Marfan's syndrome.

In Marfan's syndrome, FBNI gene of chromosome 15 is mutated, responsible for encoding fibrillin I; inherited by autosomal dominant. Clinically presents with defect in: (i) Cardiovascular tree, (ii) suspensory ligament of lens, (iii) soft and skeletal tissue defects

Indications for surgery in Marfan's syndrome

(i) Prophylactic cardiac surgery in aneurysmal dilatation of ascending aorta or valvular dysfunction
(ii) Eye surgery for retinal detachment and lens dislocation
(iii) Skeletal surgery for lordosis and scoliosis, pectus defect
(iv) Pleurodesis for penumothorax (β blockers given to retard dilatation of aorta).

SAQ 8 What is Ehlers-Danlos syndrome (EDS)?

EDS is characterised by:

(i) Hypermobile joint (ii) Skin laxity (iii) Vascular fragility
Here there is defect in collagen type I, III, V. Death is common due to rupture of blood vessels.

SAQ 9 How a rheumatoid arthritis may present?

It may present with:

(i) Arthritis
(ii) Vasculitis
(iii) Sicca syndrome
(iv) Scleritis
(v) Pulmonary fibrosis
(vi) Pleurisy
(vii) Pericarditis

LAQ 10 Mention in brief pathology of RA.

(i) Strong association with HLA-DR_4 immune response gene
(ii) IgM rheumatoid factor is present in most of the patient
(iii) Hypertrophy of synovium
(iv) Activated macrophage destructs cartilage

(v) Cartilage pannus
(vi) Growth of new vessels
(vii) Bony erosion
(viii) Oesteopenia

SAQ 11 Name the drugs of RA.

(i) NSAID particularly COX_2 inhibitors
(ii) Low dose methotrexate 10–25 mg weekly
(iii) Sulfasalazine 1g BD
(iv) Penicillamine
(v) Chloroquine

SAQ 12 Name some renal bone diseases.

In CRF, there may be associated osteomalacia and chronic secondary hyperparathyroidism.

SAQ 13 What do you mean by seronegative arthritis?

In seronegative arthritis, there is RA negativity with different groups of joints, viz. sacroiliac and spine. Generally affects capsules and insertions of tendons and ligaments (enthesiopathy).

SAQ 14 What is reactive arthritis?

In reactive arthritis, there is asymmetrical joint involvement (large) usually triggered by *Chlamydia, Shigella, Campylobacter, Yersinia* infection with severe joint tenderness, effusion, erythema. Non-articular manifestations are conjunctivitis, circinate balantitis. Maybe recurrent or persistant, self-limiting but may develop sacroilitis, HLA-B27 positive. It is sterile arthopathy.

LAQ 15 Mention the salient features of SLE.

(i) Autoimmune arthritis
(ii) Involvement of multiple systems
(iii) Non-organ specific autoantibodies with nuclear components (antinuclear and antidouble stranded DNA antibodies) may be positive for IgM rheumatoid factor

(iv) There may be renal involvement
(v) Joint involvement
(vi) Malar rash
(vii) Photosensitivity
(viii) Mouth ulcer
(ix) Discord scarring skin lesions
(x) Serositis (pleurisy and pericarditis)
(xi) Seizure
(xii) Psychosis
(xiii) Haemolytic anaemia
(xiv) False positive test for syphilis

SAQ 16 What is psoriatic arthritis?

Ten per cent of psoriatic patient may develop arthritis like RA or reactive arthritis.

SAQ 17 What is ankylosing spondylitis?

The features of ankylosing spondylitis are:

(i) Mainly affects axial skeleton
(ii) Generally associated with HLA-B27
(iii) Sacroilitis
(iv) There is progressive pain, stiffness and restrictive movements due to inflammation; fibrosis and ossification
(v) Generally affects in second decades
(vi) Treated by NSAID or DMARD (disease modifying antirheumatic drugs)

SAQ 18 What is enteropathic arthritis?

The important features of enteropathic arthritis are:

(i) Generally associated with Crohn's disease or ulcerative colitis
(ii) Generally involves lower limbs
(iii) Not associated with HLA-B27 and exacerbation of bowel disease
(iv) Generally non-erosive

SAQ 19 What are the important radiological findings of osteoarthritis?

(i) Juxta-articular sclerosis
(ii) Joint space narrowing
(iii) Marginal osteophytes

LAQ 20 What are the causes of hyperuricaemia?

It may be grouped into:

Increase uric acid production

- Idiopathic
- Malignancy, blood dyscrasia, psoriasis
- Increased purine intake

Impaired uric acid excretion

- Idiopathic CRF
- Diuretic and dehydration, starvation, diabetic ketoacidosis, surgery
- Drugs (cyclosporin, low dose aspirin)

SAQ 21 Name some crystal arthropathies.

(i) Mono-sodium urate associated gout.
(ii) Calcium pyrophosphate dehydrate with pyrophosphate arthropathy
(iii) Calcium hydroxyapatite with calcium tendonitis

Generally they have a genetic basis.

SAQ 22 Name some drugs used for gout.

(i) Cochicine
(ii) NSAID
(iii) Allopurinol
(iv) Probenecid
(v) Sulphinpyrazone
(vi) Corticosteroid
(viii) Benzbromarone

SAQ 23 What is osteoporosis?

In osteoporosis, bone resorption predominates over bone replacement.

SAQ 24 What is Paget's disease?

Paget's disease may be asymptomatic or present with bowing of tibia, spinal deformity; enlargement of skull. X-ray shows abnormal trabecular architecture with bony enlargement. Acid and alkaline phosphatase increased. Rarely turns osteosarcoma: pathological fracture may occur. May be associated with CCF, spinal stenosis, deafness.

42 The Foot

SAQ 1 Name the different congenital deformities of foot.

1. **Talipes** (a) **Talipes equinus**: Walks on toes (b) **Talipes calcaneus**: Walks on heels (c) **Talipes varus**: Walks on outer border (d) **Talipes valgus**: Walks on medial border	
2. **Talipes equinovarus**: Consisting of equinus, varus (inversion), abduction	Presents with transverse crease in medial side of sole; collosites and bursea on lateral side when patient walks. Treatment should start within 24 hours of birth with techniques of strapping, taping, splinting or plastering for 3 months. Stretching of midfoot should be avoided otherwise surgical correction
3. **Pes planus** (flatfoot): Flattening of longitudinal arch	May be congenital, traumatic, relaxed, rigid or spasmodic (contraction of peroneal muscle). For diagnosis look at medial side of foot and prints examining soles of shoes.
4. **Transverse flatfoot**: Transverse arch is dropped	Patient unable to raise metatarsal heads from grounds by pressing down toes.
5. **Pes cavus** (clawfoot): High arch foot with dorsiflexion or dorsal subluxation of metatarsophalangeal joint and plantar flexion of interphalangeal joints.	Presents in early adolescence Treated with appropriate shoes and surgery for soft tissue for mobile deformities.

LAQ 2 What is hallux valgus?

It is lateral deviation of the big toe. Common in female due to narrower footwear. Generally associated with:

(i) Exostosis
(ii) Bunion inflamed adventitious bursae
(iii) Osteoarthritis
(iv) Overriding or underriding of second toe by first.

Conservative treatment by different types of shoes is unsatisfactory. Operative treatments are:

(a) Removal of bunion
(b) Keller's operation, i.e. excision arthroplasty of the base of proximal phalanx
(c) Mayo's operation, i.e. excision of first metatarsal's head.

SAQ 3 Write short notes on: hallux rigidus, hammer toes, claw toes, Mortons's metatarsalgia, plantar fasciitis.

1. Hallux rigidus	It is painful and stiff metatarsophalangeal joint of great toe. Treated by fitting metatarsal bar or Keller's operation
2. Hammer toes	Hyperextension of metatarsophalangeal and distal interphalangeal joint and flexion of the proximal interphalangeal joint of second, third and fourth toes. Treated by correcting cause, corrective splints; corn plaster. Orthrodesis of proximal interphalangeal joints with extensor tenotomy; and dorsal capsulotomy of metatarsophalangeal joint.
3. Claw toes	It differs from hammer toe that toe pad does not contact ground and therefore increased proportion of body weight is carried by corresponding metatarsal head.
4. Morton's metatarsalgia	Here neuroma of interdigital nerve develops between metatarsal of inter digital nerves head due to nerve compression. Treated by excision of bursa
5. Plantar fasciitis	Here there is local tenderness under heal due to unknown etiology. (Maybe tear of plantar fascia; gonococcal or non-specific arthritis. Treated by rest: fitting rubber heels or insole. If not effective 25 mg hydrocortisone and 1 ml of 1% procaine injected locally.

LAQ 4 What are the different causes of pain in the foot?

Pain in foot

Front foot or metatarsalgia

- Transverse flat foot
- Morton's metatarsalgia

Mid-foot or foot strain

Pain in heel

- Fracture or disease of calcaneus
- Retrocalcaneal bursitis
- Policeman heel (infracalcaneal bursitis)
- Plantar fasciitis.

43 Osteomyelitis

SAQ 1 What is osteomyelitis?

It is infection of bone with all of its components. It may be of following types:

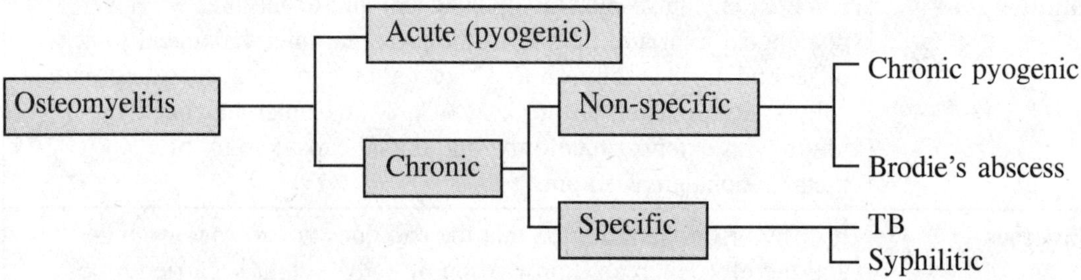

LAQ 2 Describe the pathology of osteomyelitis.

Predisposition factor: Low resistance power, septic focus

Precipitating factor: Trauma

In children, it starts in metaphysis. In adult start as primary periostitis as there is no metaphysis. It develops in following stages.

Suppuration	Necrosis	New bone formation	Soft tissue involvement
Starts as abscess in metaphysic, comes towards periosteum spreads to subperiosteal bone and shaft, may brust to soft tissues.	Diaphysis is involved, necrosis starts due to narrowing of vessels, thrombosis. Bone becomes dead producing **Sequestrum.**	Osteoblast starts forming new bone called **Involucrum.** Pus may come out of opening called **Cloaca**	Abscess may come out of cloaca to the surface.

SAQ 3 What are the different types of sequestrum?

(i) **Coralliform**: One surface smooth, another irregular like coral.
(ii) **Feathery**: Small thin in tuberculosis.
(iii) **Ivory**: Thick, hard and dense in syphilis.

(iv) **Coloured sequestrum**: Sequestrum exposed to atmosphere (tibia and fibula) are balck due to iron combining H_2S of atmosphere.
(v) **Ring sequestrum**: Formed in amputation stump.

SAQ 4 What is Brodie's abscess?

Chronic pyogenic osteomyelitis occurring insidiously due to either low virulence organism or quick control of infection but the localised organism is dormant.

SAQ 5 What are the complications of osteomyelitis?

Complications of osteomyelitis are:

General

- Toxaemia
- Septicaemia
- Bacteremia
- Pyaemia
- Amyloidosis

Local

(i) Subperiosteal abscess
(ii) Involving neighbouring joints
(iii) Pathological fracture
(iv) Deformity
(v) Chronic osteomyelitis

LAQ 6 How will you treat osteomyelitis?

Treatment of osteomyelitis

General

- Rest
- Analgesic, antipyretic
- Blood for C/S
- Antibiotics

Local

- Rest
- Drainage

Treatment of chronic osteomyelitis

If there is no sequestrum

Conservative with immobilization and antibiotics.

If there is sequestrum

Sequestromy and saucerisation to avoid recurrence

LAQ 7 What is Perthes' disease?

Perthes' disease is crushing osteochondritis affecting ossific nucleus of femoral head. It causes a vascular necrosis of ossific nucleus of femoral head.

The possible reasons are:

- Trauma
- Dysplasia
- General
- Faulty blood supply
- Metabolic or nutritional
- Infection
- Aseptic embolism

	Stage of avascular necrosis	Stage of regeneration	Stage of late-stages
Cl. features	Head fails to grow but cartilaginous portion grows.	Regeneration of head	Permanent flattening of head
X-ray	Small head; sclerosed flattened, fragmented with wider joint space.	Neck rarefied, widened, coxa vora. Acetabulum shows altered density.	Flat head with osteo-arthritis and presence of osteophytes.

SAQ 8 How to treat Perthes' disease?

Conservative: Avoid weight bearing, caliper, or crutches or by Thomas bed knee splint and splint on abduction.

Operative:

1. Drilling to vascularize head
2. Making rent on cavity and filling it with bony chips
3. Osteotomy to correct coxa vara.

LAQ 9 Describe in brief the pathology of joint tuberculosis.

Generally secondary, common in children (except wrist in adults)

Onset (i) **Primary type:** Starts with synovial membrane.
(ii) **Secondary type:** Starts in bone, then involves synovial membrane.

Stages:

Stage of synovitis	Stage of arthritis	Stage of bone destruction
Synovial membrane oedematous, hypertrophied, joint swells; synovial membrane rich in fibrin and melon seed bodies which are fibrin seeds.	Erosion in cartilage starts, formation of granular tissues and destruction of articular surface.	Bone is destroyed and **rarefying osteitis** ligaments and capsule undergoes softening, cold abscess makes way to surface or muscles.

SAQ 10 What is hydrops and carries sicca?

Hydrops: Here more synovial fluid is formed than hypertrophy of synovial membrane.

Carries sicca: Common in shoulder where muscles are atrophied

LAQ 11 Describe the clinical features of tuberculosis of hip joint.

Common below 10 years of age, starting at posteroinferior surface of neck femur Babcock's triangle, acetabular rim or head of the femur.

Presents with: (i) Pain increasing with movement (ii) Limping (iii) Constitution symptoms (fever, weight loss, night fever)

Different stages are as follows:

Stage of synovitis	Stage or arthritis	Stage of bone destruction
Flexion, abduction, external rotation, tilting down of pelvis towards affected side, lumbar lordosis, joint movements restricted	Flexion, adduction, internal roration, tilting towards opposite side: lumbar scoliosis, painful joint, muscle spasm around joint	Head strikes centre or posterior roof of acetabulum depending upon muscle pull (wondering acetabulum) true shortening, cold abscess or tubercular sinus may be found

LAQ 12 Describe the principle of treatment of TB of hip joint.

Tb hip is treated as following:

Stage of recumbency

Treated by immobilization and ATD.

Stage of ambulation with support

Movement allowed without weight bearing

Permanent treatment in healing stage

1. Subtrochanteric osteotomy
2. Arthrodesis (fixing joint from outside without opening)
   a. Iliofemoral;
   b. Ischeofemoral;
3. Intra-articular arthrodesis are considered for deformity correction
3. Gridlestone's arthroplasty

SAQ 13 What is triple displacement of knee joint?

In case of TB knee degeneration of cruciate ligament, muscle spasm producing flexion; external rotation and posterior subluxation called triple displacement.

44 Bone Tumours

SAQ 1 How are the bones composed of?

Bones are composed of tissues of mesenchyma.

SAQ 2 From what sources, tumours of bones may arise?

It may arise from bone, cartilage, fat, endothelium and fibrous tissues.

SAQ 3 Classify bone tumours according to source.

Source	Benign	Malignant
Bone forming tumour	• Osteoid osteoma • Osteoma	• Osteosarcoma • Periosteal osteosarcoma • Dedifferentiated osteosarcoma
Cartilage forming tumours	• Enchondroma • Osteochondroma • Periosteal enchondroma • Chondroblastoma • Chondromixoid fibroma	• Chondrosarcoma • Mesenchymal chondrosarcoma • Dedifferentiated chondrosarcoma • Mixoid chondrosarcoma • Clear cell Chondrosarcoma
Fat cell		• Liposarcoma
Fibrous tumours	• Non-ossifying fibroma • Fibrous dysplasia • Desmoplastic fibroma	• Fibrosarcoma
Vascular tumours	• Haemangioma	• Haemangioendothelioma • Haemangiopericytoma • Angiosarcoma

(Contd.)

Source	Benign	Malignant
Giant cells **Marrow tumour**	Giant cell tumour	• Malignant giant cell tumour • Ewing's sarcoma • Peripheral neuroepithelioma • Lymphoma • Myeloma
Other varieties		• Parchondroma • Adamantinoma • Mesenchymoma • Undifferentiated sarcoma • Histocytoma

LAQ 4 How to diagnose bone tumours?

High degree of suspicion for early referral is important which is achieved by:

(i) History and examination
- Duration
- Pain
- Mass

(ii) Investigations
- Radiograph
- Nuclear bone scan
- CT
- MRI
- PET
- Thallium scans

SAQ 5 Mention the principles of management of bone tumours.

Bone tumours are staged by biopsy (immuno, histochemical, histological)

- Surgery for benign tumours
- Surgery with chemotherapy with radiotherapy for Ewing's tumour.
- Chemotherapy prior to surgery (neoadjuvants)

SAQ 6 What are the risk factors of fracture of metastatic bone tumours?

These are:

(i) Osteolytic lesion
(ii) Two-thirds of bone destruction
(iii) Pain with activity
(iv) Intertrochanteric lesion

SAQ 7 What are the salient features of the multiple myeloma?

This common primary malignancy of bone presents with:

(i) Bony pain, anaemia
(ii) Age over 65 years
(iii) Raised ESR, Bence Jones proteins
(iv) Monoclonal gammopathy.

SAQ 8 Describe the radiological findings of Ewing's sarcoma, osteosarcoma.

Ewing's sarcoma: Common in paediatric age group radiologically presents with permeative destruction of bones onion ring type.

Osteosarcoma: Common in 9–16 years of age around knee and upper arm with periosteal elevation called sunray type of spiculation.

Extraosseous components of tumour can be seen on MRI.

LAQ 9 Classify bony tumours according to Graham-Apley.

(i) It may be benign; malignant; intermediate
(ii) According to origin of cells: From framework cells; resident cells; invader cells
(iii) Graham-Apley classification:

- **Benign**
  - From framework
    - Osteoma
    - Chondroma
    - Chondroblastoma
    - Osteochondroma
  - From resident cells
    - Fibroma
    - Lipoma (rare)
    - Haemangioma
    - Aneurysmal bone cyst
- **Malignant**
  - Framework
    - Osteogenic sarcoma
    - Chondrosarcoma
    - Fibrosarcoma
  - Resident cells
    - Ewing's tumour
    - Multiple myeloma
  - Secondary invader carcinoma
- **Osteoclastoma**
- **Chondroma**

SAQ 10 What is Bryant's triangle; Nelaton's line; Schoemaker's line?

Bryant's triangle	Nelaton's line	Schoemaker's line
Patient lies dorsally, triangle formed by: (a) one line joining ASIS to bed; tip of greater trochanter to join 1st line; and line joining ASIS to greater trochanter The shortening of 2nd line compared to same of other side indicates upward elevation of greater trochanter. 3rd line helps to determine AP displacement of trochanter.	Patient lies on sound side Line is drawn from ASIS and ischial tuberosity which generally touches tip of greater trochanter.	Line joining ASIS and greater trochanter is extended and should cross it above trochanter is extended umbilicus except in elevation of trochanter below the umbilicus
	NB: ASIS = Anterior superior iliac spine	

SAQ 11 What is Trendelenburg test?

Pelvis normally rises to opposite side, if patient stands on one leg, it drops on other side, if patient stands on diseased side the test is said to be positive.

SAQ 12 Name the fractures and dislocations which can occur with fall in out stretched hand.

(i) Fracture scaphoid
(ii) Colles' fracture
(iii) Fracture radial head
(iv) Dislocation of elbow
(v) Supracondylar fracture
(vi) Fracture humoral neck
(vii) Dislocation of shoulder.

SAQ 13 Describe the X-ray appearance of osteoclastoma.

The osteoclastoma (source is either from fibrous dysplasia or from spindle cells of bones) radiologically diagnosed by:

(i) Situated at the end of long bones, eccentric, lies transversly to long axis, with definitive line of demarcation from healthy bones, destruction of bones give soap bubble appearance, without soft tissue shadow.

(ii) If turns malignant, there will be soft tissue shadow, outline of cortex is lost, and demarcation from healthy bone lost.

Treated by surgery amputation or radiotherapy (moderately radiosensitive).

SAQ 14 What is Codman triangle?

It is found in osteogenic sarcoma (periosteal variety) where tumour is massive, periosteum lift it, and rejoins the bone little away from diaphyseal end of the tumour producing a triangle.

Base of triangle is formed by tumour, apex at a site where periosteum rejoins shaft. Codman triangle represents recreative bone.

SAQ 15 Describe the microscopic appearance and different modes of spread of osteogenic sarcoma.

The osteogenic sarcoma is pleomorphic. The different cell varieties are spindle cells, tumour and foreign body giant cells. Intracellular substances may show hyaline, fibrous, cartilaginous myxaematous, osseous even at same tumour. It contains numerous thin-walled blood vessels in which endothelial lining may be missing.

It spreads by direct, lymphatic and venous pathway.

LAQ 16 Write note on ankylosis.

Ankylosis is limitation of joint movements.

Ankylosis

- **True**
  Intraarticular lesion
  - **Fibrous**
    Bones are held by fibrous tissue
  - **Bony**
    Bones are held by bony tissue
- **False**
  Contracture of periarticular soft tissue:
  - By skin and subcutaneous tissue (burn)
  - Muscle and tendon (VIC)
  - Fascia (Dupytren's contracture)
  - Ligaments (due to immobilisation)
  - Bone (ankylosing spondylitis, myositis ossification)

SAQ 17 Mention the position of ease and optimum position of following joints.

	Hip	Knee	Ankle	Shoulder	Elbow	Wrist
Position of ease	Flexion Abduction External	Flexion	Plantar flexion and inversion	Abduction	Flexion	Plantar flexion
Optimum position	20° flexion, 10° abduction	5–10° flexion	Neutral to dorsal and Plantar flexion	70° Abduction 30° front of coronal plane	90° for clerk 160°for labour	15–20° dorsi-flexion

By position of ease, we mean, position in which maximum position within joint space.

By optimum position, we mean, the position in which maximum function of the joint can be done.

45

Fracture and Dislocations

SAQ 1 What is fracture?

Fracture is discontinuity in continuity of bones.

LAQ 2 What are the important causes of fractures?

The important causes are:

(i) Age: More common in active age and in elderly (osteoporosis)

(ii) Violence:

- (a) Energy of trauma ($E = \frac{1}{2} \times mass \times velocity^2$)
- (b) Direct violence
- (c) Indirect violence (fall in out stretched hand produces clavicular fracture)
- (d) Stress
- (e) Muscular contraction, e.g. fracture of patella and greater tuberosity of humerus; convulsions

LAQ 3 What are the types of fracture?

Types of fracture depend upon types of injury; age of patient. It may be:

(i) **Displaced or undisplaced fractures**

(ii) **Transverse:** Passes transversely; union is slow.

(iii) **Oblique and spiral:** Caused by twisting force: quick union.

(iv) **Impacted**: One segments driven into another, stable should be immobilized; union is quick.

(v) **Comminuted fracture:** Bone broken into several segments by direct injury, unstable and difficult to retain in position.

(vi) **Butterfly fracture:** One triangular butterfly segment lies between bones.

(vii) **Segmental fracture:** Bone broken into several segments.

(viii) **Avulsion fracture:** Caused by sudden contraction of muscle.

(ix) **Compression fracture:** Caused by compressive force common in lumbar spine.

(x) **Green stick fracture:** Periosteal continuity is maintained in one side, but other side is broken like bamboo stick. Common in children.

(xi) **Compound fracture:** In compound fracture, sites communicate to environment, prone to infection.

(xii) **Epiphyseal fracture:** Involves epiphyseal plate of long bone.

SAQ 4 Classify epiphyseal fractures.

According to Salter-Harris, the epiphyseal fracture may be of following grades:

Grade 1: Small crack along metaphyseal side of epiphyseal plate

Grade 2: Fracture line travels along metaphyseal side of plate and breaks it, commonest with best prognosis.

Grade 3: Fracture line crosses from metaphysis to epiphysis

Grade 4: Fracture line travels along the distal epiphyseal side of the growth plate. It deviates into the epiphysis itself out of articular surface.

Grade 5: Severe crush of epiphyseal plate.

SAQ 5 How fractures are classified internationally?

1. The first number relates to bone (viz. 1 for humerus; radius and ulna 2)
2. Position number is followed by severity
3. Proximal fracture type1; distal fractures type 2.
4. A, B, C indicate extra-articular; partial articular and articular
5. Diaphyseal fractures type 2: (a) A is simple; (b) B is butterfly; (c) C is comminuted

SAQ 6 Mention the steps of fracture healing.

Fracture heals as follows:

Stage of haematoma

↓

Formation of haematoma

↓

Formation of callus

↓

Further development of callus

↓

Deposition of new bones

↓

Remodelling of new bones

SAQ 7 What are the disadvantages of international classification of fracture?

(i) It is difficult to memorise
(ii) It does not give mode of treatment and prognosis
(iii) It does not give clue for displacements

SAQ 8 What are the different varieties of callus formation?

The different varieties of callus formations are:

(i) Normal amount of callus formation
(ii) Minimal callus formation but with union
(iii) Non-union with excessive callus formation
(iv) No callus with fibrous union

SAQ 9 How to diagnose fracture?

(i) History, (ii) pain and tenderness, (iii) abnormal mobility, (iv) radiologically

SAQ 10 What is the average time for union for following bones of upper and lower limbs?

Upper limbs		*Lower limbs*	
Bones	*Time*	*Bones*	*Time*
Clavicle	3–4 weeks	Femur	10–12 weeks
Humerus	6–8 weeks	Tibia	8–12 weeks
Radius shaft	8–10 weeks	Fibula	8–10 weeks
Lower end	6–8 weeks	Tarsals	6–8 weeks
Ulna	8–10 weeks	Metatarsal	4–6 weeks
Carpal	6–8 weeks	Calcaneum	8–12 weeks
Metacarpals	3 weeks		

LAQ 11 What are the defects of bone union?

(i) Delayed union due to
- Bones with poor blood supply
- Comminuated fracture
- Intervening soft tissue
- Fracture of one of paired bones
- Imperfect reduction and immobilization
- Infection
- Over traction
- Inadequate fixation

(ii) Non-union due to
- Separate segments
- Sclerosis
- Inadequate callus
- Pseudo-joint

(iii) Malunion

(iv) Shortening

LAQ 12 Mention the different complications of fracture.

Complications of fracture

- **General**
  - Tetanus
  - Gangrene
- **Visceral injuries**
  - Chest
  - Abdomen, etc.
- **Local**
  - **Skin**
    - Abrasion
    - Laceration
  - **Muscle**
    - Rupture
    - Myositis-ossificans
    - Tendon rupture
  - **Vessels**
    - Haemorrhage
    - Thrombosis
    - Embolism
    - Atrophy
  - **Bone**
    - Non-delayed or malunion
    - Osteoporosis
  - **Joint**
    - Degeneration
    - Arthritis

SAQ 13 Define dislocation subluxation and sprain.

Dislocation: It is complete disruption of joints with articular surface displaced.
Subluxation: Disruption of joints without articular surface disruption.
Sprain: Here joints are stretched involving ligaments and capsule with partial rupture

SAQ 14 What are the indications of open reduction?

(i) Open fracture
(ii) Fracture cannot be reduced
(iii) Displaced fracture
(iv) Unstable fracture
(v) Displaced intraarticular fracture in children

LAQ 15 What do you mean by rigid and non-rigid fixation? What are the types of fixation?

Rigid fixation allows immediate loading but does not allow callus formation. Non-rigid fixation by plaster of Paris allows limited movement and callus formation is good.

Fixation may be external or internal.

Fixation can be done by:

(i) Screw
(ii) Plates (Butress, dynamic compression plates (DCP, neutralization plates)
(iii) Wires (Kapanji wires, firgure of eight wiring)
(iv) Intermedullarly nails

SAQ 16 What are the causes of joint stiffness in fracture?

Important causes of post-fracture joint stiffness are:

(i) Periarticular adhesion
(ii) Intraarticular adhesion
(iii) Muscular adhesion
(iv) Degenerative arthritis

SAQ 17 What are the important complications of tension following fracture?

(i) Avulsion fracture
(ii) Late rupture of tendons

SAQ 18 Write short note on Volkmann's ischaemic contracture (VIC).

VIC is serious complication of fracture due to arterial blood supply interference generally in upper limb in supera-condylar fracture. Interference of blood supply causes ischaemic neurosis.

Fibrosis contracture. Arterial blood supply may be interfered due to:

(i) Spasm
(ii) External pressure or kink
(iii) Thrombosis

Diagnosis:

- Impaired pulsation
- Numbness
- Discoloration
- Coldness
- Swelling

Fractures of Superior and Inferior Extremity

46

SAQ 1 What is Monteggia's fracture?

(i) Dislocation of radial head at elbow ─┐
(ii) Proximal ulnar fracture ─────────┘→ Together called Monteggia's fracture

SAQ 2 What is Galleazi fracture?

Distal radial fracture with separation of distal ulnar epiphysis. Treated with closed reduction.

LAQ 3 What is Colles' fracture?

This commonest fracture of lower end of radius within 3/4th inch of wrist joint associated with injury of the inferior radioulnar joint, relative displacement between lower articulating surfaces of radius and ulna with or without tear of medial collateral ligament of wrist, with or without avulsion of ulna.

It is generally transverse fracture, but maybe T-shaped.

Displacements are:

(i) Upwards (impaction)

(ii) Backwards

(iii) Laterally

(iv) Backwards tilt

(v) Supination of lower fragments

Clincal features: • Pain • Swelling • Limitation of movements of wrist joint • Dinner fork deformity • Tenderness of lower end of radius • Radial styloid process is either at same level of ulnar styloid process or above.

Treatment

(i) Reduction under GA
 (a) Disimpaction
 (b) Correction of backward displacement of lower fragments and lateral displacement and supination.

(ii) Immobilization by plaster extending below elbow up to knuckle with base of thumb free for 6 weeks, i.e. Colles' plastering.

(iii) Exercise

Complications

- Malunion
- OA
- Rupture of extensor pollicis longus
- Movement restriction
- Sudeck bone atrophy
- Difficulties in movement of supination and pronation is treated by excision of lower end of ulna or corrective osteotomy
- Palmar flexion limitation is corrected by osteotomy of lower radius.

SAQ 4 What is Smith's or reversed Colles' fracture?

It is transverse fracture of lower radius with forward tilt of lower segment due to fall on back of hand with flexed wrist.

SAQ 5 Write short note on scaphoid fracture.

Generally occurs through waist of scaphoid bone. Avascular necrosis of proximal fragment is common. Recent fracture is generally missed on AP view, so better diagnosed on lateral view. Anatomical snuff box tenderness is common.

Complications: • Avascular necrosis • Delayed union • Non-union • Malunion • OA

Treatment: Immobilization below elbow like Colles' fracture including proximal digits and thumb wrist in dorsiflexion with forward placing of thumb (Glass holding position for minimum 8 weeks).

LAQ 6 Classify supracondylar fracture.

Supracondylar fracture is commonest injury through lower end of humerus can be classified as follows:

Supracondylar fracture

- **Amongst children**
  - **Supracondylar fracture**
    - Posterior displacement
    - Anterior displacement
    - Green stick
  - **Medial epicondylar fracture**
    - Minimal displacement
    - Gross displacement
    - Displacement inside joint
    - Gross displacement with dislocation of elbow joint
  - **Lateral condylar fracture**
    - Lateral condylar fracture with minimal displacement
    - Lat. condylar fracture with displacement and rotation.
- **Amongst adults**
  - T- and Y-shaped fracture with intercondylar fracture
  - Fracture capitellum
  - Fracture condyles
  - Ant. and post. dislocation

SAQ 7 What is mallet finger?

This is avulsion due to sudden severe contraction of extensor tendon of the finger.

It should be treated immediately by mallet splint. The terminal interphalangeal joint is hyper-extended and proximal interphalangeal joint is flexed to 90° on table. A ½" plaster of 3–4 layer is wrapped in finger extended up to proximal phalynx for 6 weeks.

LAQ 8 What are the different types of dislocations of elbow joint?

Elbow dislocation is quite common due to indirect violence (fall in outstretched hand with elbow flexed).

Types

- **Posterior dislocation**: Commonest, radius and ulnar placed posteriorly with lateral or medial shift
- **Anterior dislocation**: Bones displaced anteriorly, olecranon process lies above condyles of humerus
- **Medial or lateral dislocation** (rare type)

LAQ 9 How the fractures of olecranon process is treated?

Olecranon fracture is due to indirect or direct injury.

Types: (i) Undisplaced fracture, (ii) displaced fracture, (iii) comminuted fracture.

Diagnosis:

- Pain
- Swelling
- Tenderness
- Painful restricted extension of elbow joint
- X-ray for confirmation

Complications: • Non-union • Osteoarthritis

Treatment

- **Conservative**
  - Immobilization with flexed elbow with dorsal slab applied on elbow flexed at 90° for 4–6 weeks
  - Immobilization in extension extending up to axilla to wireloop metacarpal heads for 4–6 weeks
- **Operative**
  - Fixation by screw or segment
  - Excision of fracture

LAQ 10 Mention the displacements of fracture of forearm bones.

Displacements are done by pronator teres, pronator quadratus, and supinator muscles.

- Fracture of upper one-third of radius Proximal supination, distal pronation stability achieved by immobilization
- Fracture of mid one-third of radius stability is achieved by immobilization in midway of prone and supination
- Fracture of lower one-third lower portion prone, proximal segment mid prone immobilized in prone

LAQ 11 Write short notes on dislocation of hip joint.

The hip joint is ball and socket joint covered by strong capsules and ligaments. Following types of dislocations may occur:

Posterior dislocation	Anterior dislocation	Central dislocation
Due to violence along long axis of femur, viz. traffic accidents. **Types** (i) Simple (ii) With fracture of acetabulum (iii) With fracture of femur head. **Diagnosis**: Leg is shorter, flexed, internally rotated with prominent greater trochanter X-ray. **Treatment**:Should be treated promptly to avoid avascular necrosis of femoral head and sciatic nerve injury. (a) Reduction under GA: (b) Post-reduction management: (i) Immobilization by skin or skeletal traction (ii) Weight bearing after 6 wks (iii) X-rays at interval to notice avascular necrosis of femur head. **Complications**: (i) Post-acetabular fracture (ii) Fracture femoral head (iii) Injury of sciatic nerve (iv) Unreduced dislocation (v) Avascular necrosis of femoral head.	Occurs due to direct injury from behind. **Diagnosis**: Limb is flexed, abducted and external rotated and by X-rays in AP and lat view. **Treatment**: Reduction under GA. Flexed thigh is internally rotated and adducted Post-reduction X-rays.	Less common, occur due to violent injury. **Types**: (i) Fracture of acetabulum without displacement (ii) Moderate and (iii) Severe intrapelvic displacement **Diagnosis**: Painful and restricted hip movement with bruise and ecchymosis. X-ray confirms. (a) **Treatment**: Fracture of acetabulum without displacement: Hamilton-Russel traction with exercise and non-weight bearing. (b) Fracture of acetabulum with displacement. Reduction under GA; Traction post-reduction X-ray and Hamilton-Russel traction for 2 months. Non-weight bearing crutches after months. Allow weight bearing after 3 months.

LAQ 12 Write note on fracture neck femur.

Common in postmenopausal osteoporotic woman. Due to twisting, sprain or pathological fracture.

Problems of fracture neck femur:

• Interruption of blood supply • Poor callus formation • Poor stability

Classification:

(i) Subcapital (commonest)
(ii) Transcervical
(iii) Basal subcapital is prone to avascular necrosis

Garden's classification:

Stage I (Incomplete without dislocation) satisfactory result with internal fixation.
Stage II (Complete without dislocation) satisfactory result with internal fixation.
Stage III (Abducted disimpacted) unstable, requires proper reduction before fixation.
Stage IV (Extreme disimpacted) excision of head with metallic prosthesis is ideally required.

Diagnosis: History: Clinical exam, X-ray.

Excision of femoral head is required for:

(i) Unstable fracture
(ii) Failure of internal fixation
(iii) Ischaemia of head

Fracture of femoral head in children and young may be due to pathological fracture or slipped epiphysis.

Treated by: (i) Plaster immobilization, (ii) Internal fixation by Knowles pin.

Postoperative management: Early ambulation but no weight bearing for 3 months and exercise.

Complications of fracture neck femur:

(i) Non-union
(ii) Asceptic avascular necrosis requires reconstructive operation
(iii) Complications of the pin.

LAQ 13 Write short note on patellar fracture.

Patella, the largest sesamoid bone, situated under quadriceps expansion may be fractured by:

(a) Direct and
(b) Indirect violence (by violent contraction of extensor muscles)
(c) Direct and indirect force

The fracture may be:

(i) Complete or incomplete
(ii) Displaced or undisplaced

Diagnosed by:

(i) History
(ii) Physical exam and X-ray

Treatment

A. Conservative for undisplaced fracture with:
   (i) Aspiration
   (ii) Compression bandage
   (iii) Application of dorsal splint and plaster cylinder for immobilization for 6 weeks
B. Surgery (preservation, total excision, partial excision and marginal excision of patella)

SAQ 14 Classify pelvic bone injury.

It may be:

- **Avulsion fracture**
- **Isolated pelvic ring fracture**
  - Fracture ileum
  - Fracture pubis
  - Fracture ischium
  - Fracture floor of acetabulum
- **Pelvic ring disruption**
  - Anterior posterior compression fracture
  - Lateral compression fracture
  - Vertical force
- **Sacrococcygeal fracture**

Bleeding injury of bladder, rectum, pelvic colon, damage to nerve may occur with pelvic bone fracture.

SAQ 15 What are the causes of sprain in cervical spine?

It generally occurs with automobile injury where head trusted forward and body backwards producing hyperflexion, hyperextension, lateral flexion or twisting

Treated by • Rest • Analgesic • Exercise • Cervical collar • Intermittent traction.

SAQ 16 What problem may arise out of fracture of axis odontoid process?

It may arise out of automobile accident, gymnastic activity, fall from height or on head. If it is displaced, it may cause spinal compression.

SAQ 17 What are the different types of fracture that may occur in cervical spine?

(i) Compression fracture of the body
(ii) Brust fracture
(iii) Fracture of lamina
(iv) Fracture of spinous process

LAQ 18 What are the different types of injuries possible in thoracolumbar region?

From T_1–T_{10} are less likely to injury:

T_{10}–T_{12} and lumbar spines are mobile and liable to injury: L_5 and sacral portion is likely to get sprain injury

Injuries in thoracolumbar spinal region

- **Simple fracture**
  - Anterior wedge compression fracture
  - Brust fracture
  - Fracture of transverse process
- **Fracture dislocation**
- **Dislocation**

SAQ 19 What are the causes of nerve pressure in spinal injuries?

- Oedema
- Haemorrhage
- Pressure by displaced segments.

Problems of Shoulder and Elbow

47

SAQ 1 What is sprengel deformity?

Here scapula is high, small and rotated and may be connected to cervical spine by omovertebral body a fibrous or bony bar, due to failure of normal descent of scapula.

LAQ 2 What is frozen shoulder?

Here due to unknown etiology, rotator interval, supraspinatous, subscapularis and subscapularis of shoulder are affected causing painful shoulder. Common in female above 50 in diabetics, heart or thyroid disease. It has three stages.

- **(i) Stage I (painful phase):** With severe pain at night may be unrelieved by analgesics (2–9 month).
- **(ii) Stage II (stiffening phase):** Pain gradually reduces but reduction of movement (lasts 4–12 months)
- **(iii) Stage III (stage of thawing)** movement gradually improves.

Treatment

- (i) Corticosteroid
- (ii) Active and passive mobilization
- (iii) Surgery for prolonged stiffness (arthroscopic distension or open release of rotator interval)

SAQ 3 What is calcific tendonitis?

In calcific tendonitis, calcium is deposited in supraspinatous, presents with pain on anterolateral aspect of shoulder with activity. It may be self-limiting or

Treated with:

- (i) Analgesic
- (ii) Physiotherapy
- (iii) Subacromial injections of corticosteroid
- (iv) Surgery
  - (a) Excision of calcific deposits
  - (b) Arthroscopy with subacromial decompression

LAQ 4 What is tennis elbow?

Occurs due to unaccustomed activity involving active extension and supination of wrist, producing partial tear and inflammation of extensor carpi brevis causing pain around elbow. Diagnosed by history, clinically, ultrasound, MRI.

Treatment

(i) Avoid precipitating cause
(ii) Analgesia
(iii) Local hydrocortisone
(iv) Physiotherapy
(v) Occasionally surgery (excision of abnormal tissue)

SAQ 5 What is golfer's elbow?

Here common flexor origin of medial epicondyl is involved. Diagnosed by history, clinical exam, ultrasound, MRI. Treated medically or surgically.

SAQ 6 Write short note on loose bodies of elbow.

Etiology: OA, osteochondritis

Clinical presentation: Pain around elbow, lock elbow

Treated by: Orthoscopic removal of loose bodies.

LAQ 7 What is olecranon bursitis?

Inflammation of olecranon bursa, presents with red, warm, swollen, painful, confined to back of elbow due to chemical inflammation.

Treated with:

(i) Rest
(ii) Ice
(iii) NSAID
(iv) Compress and dressing
(v) Antibiotics
(vi) If due to calcified nodule surgical excision should be avoided.

LAQ 8 Write short note on fracture of clavicle.

Cause: Common in male than female 2.5:1 due to indirect (fall in out stretched hand) or direct trauma. Site is mid-shaft with overlapping and lateral third.

Treatment

(i) Conservatively by limb rest with broad arm sling.
(ii) Figure of eight bandage overlapping is reduced by pressure by flexed knee from behind in between shoulder blades.
(iii) Open reduction of lateral ends fracture with plate fixation.
(iv) Internal fixation with bone graft for non-union symptomatic fracture. Look for neurovascular compression and regular tightening of figure of eight bandage is required.

SAQ 9 Write short note on acrominoclavicular disruption.

Caused by trauma, common in young male associated with dislocation of clavicle and superior subluxation.

Treated by broad arm sling conservatively. Lateral end clavicular displacement requires surgical reconstruction.

LAQ 10 Write short note on shoulder dislocation.

Shoulder joint is less stable compared to many other because of shallow genoid fossa's articular surface circumference of head of humerus. Dislocation occurs due to fall in out stretched hand, tetanus, epilepsy or by direct injury.

Types

(i) Anterior dislocation head of humerus displaced under subcoracoid process
(ii) Posterior dislocation
(iii) Inferior dislocation (hyperabduction injury). Head goes to infraglenoid position.

Diagnosis

(i) History
(ii) Unable to lift affected arm
(iii) Comparision with normal arm
(iv) X-ray confirms diagnosis:

Treatment

- **Anterior dislocation**
  - **Kocher's method**
    - (a) Traction
    - (b) Lateral rotation
    - (c) Adduction
    - (d) Internal rotation
  - **Hippocratic method**
    - Both done under GA
- **Posterior dislocation**
  - Done under GA
  - (a) Traction on arm
  - (b) Adduction
  - (c) External rotation
  - (d) Internal rotation
- **Inferior dislocation**
  - Traction in abduction
  - Gentle adduction of the limb

After treatment of reduction: (i) X-ray (AP and lateral); immobilization in triangular bandage for 3 weeks. Note any nerve lesion.

Complications: Nerve injury, muscle injury (supraspinatous, biceps), recurrence, bony injury (greater tuberosity, neck of humerus).

LAQ 11 Write short note on fracture neck of humerus.

Common in osteoporotic menopausal woman. Falling in out stretched hand. Fracture may be impacted, separated or angulated (adduction or abduction with or without impaction).

Diagnosis: Swelling, pain, tenderness, restricted joint movement and by X-ray (two views).

Treatment

- **Impacted fracture**
  - Disimpact if grossly angulated otherwise simple collar and cuff with exercise of fingers
  - Shoulder spica of 3–4 weeks selected in cases in children
- **Displaced fracture**
  - Reduction under GA immobilization.
  - Traction or open reduction

48 Spine and Spinal Cord Injury

SAQ 1 What are the different mechanisms of spinal cord injury?

It may occur in:

(i) Acute flexion causing long axis stretch
(ii) Nipping of cord in between lamina and fractured body
(iii) Protrusion of disc in flexion movement causing anterior compression.

SAQ 2 How long the spinal cord extends?

In adult, it extends below the body of 1st lumbar vertebra.

LAQ 3 What is spinal shock or spinal concussion? How it manifests?

Sudden long axis stretch of spinal cord following flexion causes displacement of supporting tissues of nerve fibres and disturbances of nerve conduction.

Nipping of the cord between lamina and displaced vertebrae may cause transverse contusion with bruising. Massive haemorrhage of spinal cord called haematomyelia.

Clinical features: Loss of sensastion below lesion; ascending of paralysis indicates ascending oedema.

The spinal cord contusion can be categorized into:

(a) Stage of spinal shock
(b) Return of activities
(c) Stage of septic complication (like bedsore, pneumonia or urinary infection can occur)

Cervical spines have higher mobility with little strength so they are easily prone to fracture and dislocation to minor injuries, compared to dorsal and lumbar spine which are stronger, required more forces for fracture and dislocation.

LAQ 4 What is spina bifida?

Gap in posterior wall of vertebral column due to developmental defects. It may be:

A. **Spina bifida cystica** (protrusion of meninges through the gap. Its different varieties are:
   (a) Meningocele, i.e. meninges containing CSF protrude
   (b) Meningomyelocele: Meninges and spinal cord protrude

(c) Syringomyelocele: Meninges, spinal cord and central canal protrudes
(d) Myelocele: Along with vertebral defect posterior part of the cord is also not developed

B. **Spina bifida occulta**: Here there is no protrusion of spinal cord.

LAQ 5 Define the following spinal deformities (scoliosis, kyphosis, lordosis).

- **Scoliosis, i.e. lateral curvature of spine**
  - Mobile
    - **Postural** : In schoolgoing child
    - **Compensatory**
      - Torticolis
      - Pneumo-nectomy
      - PID
      - Short leg
  - Fixed
    - **Idiopathic**
    - Congenital
    - **Paralytic**
      - Polio
      - Neuro-fibromatosis
- **Kyphosis, i.e. anterior bending**
  - Round back
    - Osteoporosis
    - Paget's disease, hemivertebra
  - Hump back
    - Caries
    - Carcinoma
    - Fracture
- **Lordosis, i.e. posterior bending like lord**
  - Pregnancy
  - Ricket
  - CDH
  - Short tendo-Achilles

LAQ 6 Mention the different tumours of vertebral column and spinal canal.

- **Tumours**
  - **Vertebral column**
    - **Benign**
      - Chondroma
      - Osteoma
      - Fibroma
    - **Malignant**
      - **Primary**
        - Sarcoma
        - Neurofibroma
      - **Secondary**
    - **Extradural**
      - Lipoma
      - Meningoma
  - **Intraspinal**
    - **Intra-medullary**
      - Gilioma
      - Meningioma
    - **Extra-medullary**
      - Neurofibroma

SAQ 7 What is ankylosing spondylitis?

In this crippling disease, which is more in male, there is:

(i) HLA-B27 association.
(ii) Ankylosis of central articulation due to calcification of ligaments and capsules of joints.
(iii) Sacroiliac spine from lumbar region hip, costal joint and patient is double bent enventually.
(iv) Bamboo spine deformity.

Treated by: NSAID, Postural exercise, osteotomy of spine.

LAQ 8 What is caries spine? What complications it may produce?

Tuberculosis of spine is called ***caries spine*** or ***Pott's disease*** involves body of the vertebra. It is always secondary and reaches the spine by bloodstream. May lead to following complications.

Deformity of spinal cord	Spreading of cold abscess	Pott's paraplegia
• Kyphosis • Gibbus • Scoliosis	• Paraplegia • Pre- and paravertebral abscess • Pharyngeal abscess • Abscess in mediastinum • Abscess in lateral lumbo-costal arch • Median arcuate ligament • Psoas abscess • Abscess popliteal fossa • Petit's triangle of thigh • Ischeorectal abscess.	• Due to cold abscess, caeseous mass and tuberculours granulation tissue. **Types**: (Early onset) (i) **Type-I** recovers within 6 months of treatment **Type-II** does not recover within 6 months (ii) Late onset due to fibrosis; thrombosis and reactivation of lesion

49 Head Injury

SAQ 1 What are the layers of scalp?

Scalp has following layers:

S = Skin
C = Subcutaneous tissue
A = Aponeurosis
L = Loose areolar tissue
P = Periosteum

SAQ 2 What is Wen?

These are retention sebaceous cysts of the scalp often multiple; may cause baldness if it interferes with blood supply.

SAQ 3 What is cirsoid aneurysm?

Capillary naevi in skin underneath which abnormal arteries communicate directly with distended veins. Branches of temporal artery are affected. Treated by extirpation.

SAQ 4 Why there is excessive bleeding is scalp wound and why it heals quickly?

Because blood vessels cannot contract as it lies within aponeurosis. Rich blood supply heals it quickly.

> Scalp is closed in two layers: Aponeurosis to aponeurosis and skin to skin

SAQ 5 Define microcephaly, oxycephaly and meningocele.

Microcephaly: May be congenital or due to premature synostosis. May cause agenesis of brain or imbecility.

Oxycephaly: Egg-shaped skull due to premature obliteration of sutures.

Meningocele: Protrusion of a pouch of dura mater through skull.

SAQ 6 What complications may arise in osteomyelitis of skull?

- Infective thrombosis of emissary veins
- Extradural abscess
- Subdural abscess
- Brain abscess
- Meningitis

SAQ 7 What is the pathology of injury of brain?

(i) Diffuse neuronal lesions during impact due to displacement and distortion of cerebral tissues.
(ii) Oedema, intracranial haemorrhage, etc. are secondary changes take time to develop.

SAQ 8 What are the aims of carniosynostosis surgery?

- To increase skull volume
- Improve airways
- Cosmetic purpose

SAQ 9 Describe the different displacements of brain injury.

Lateral displacement not possible due to falx septum in midline. Anteroposterior riding movment within CSF space occurs as it is suspended by superior cerebral veins.

SAQ 10 What is cerebral concussion, contusion and laceration?

Cerebral concussion: Here brain is slightly stretched with temporary paralysis of physiological functions without structural damage with complete recovery.

Cerebral contusion: Severe stretching , with rupture of fibres, incomplete recovery. Death occurs independent of intracranial pressure.

Cerebral laceration: Brain surface is torn with effusion of blood in CSF plus internal changes as seen in contusion.

SAQ 11 What is Hutchison's pupil?

1st stage: Pupil of affected side constricts and other side is normal
2nd stage: Effected side pupil dilates and other side constricts.
3rd stage: Both side pupils are dilated.

SAQ 12 What are the signs of pontine haemorrhage?

- Pyrexia
- Pin point fixed pupil
- Paralysis

SAQ 13 What are the signs and symptoms of raised intracranial pressure?

(i) Headache (worse in morning due to vasodilation, hypoventilation due to CO_2 retention)
(ii) Nausea
(iii) Vomiting
(iv) Papilloedema

SAQ 14 What are the different options of treatment of raised ICP?

(i) **Drugs:** Steroids, manitol, barbiturate, frusemide
(ii) Hypothermia
(iii) Removal of intracranial mass
(iv) Ventilation
(v) Ventriculotomy for CSF drainage

SAQ 15 What are the different mechanisms of fracture of a skull?

It may occur due to:
(i) Compression
(ii) Local indentation
(iii) Tangential injury

LAQ 16 Mention in brief the principle of closed head injury.

(i) Quick clinical examination and determine serverity
(ii) Nursing care
(iii) Nasal feeding
(iv) Observation for complications
(v) Treatment of skull fracture
(vi) Posture (Coleman position)
(vii) Tracheostomy
(viii) Catheterization
(ix) Drugs paraldehyde for restless patient; mannitol (IV); diuretics
(x) Hypothermia improves prognosis
(xi) Therapeutic lumbar puncture on alternate days.

LAQ 17 What are the different types of traumatic intracranial haemorrhage?

It may be:

Subcortical	Extradural	Subdural
Due to arterial or rupture of central artery. **Clinical features**: Cerebral compression and epileptic fits and focal features.	Torn of internal maxillary or anterior meningeal vessels or due to injury of anterior and posterior branches of middle cerebral artery. **Clinical features**: Short initial period of concussion; lucid interval, then confusion change in level of consciousness, pupil dilated, bruising and fracture should be treated earlier with operation.	Caused by rupture of vessels passing cerebral hemisphere to venous sinus. **Clinical features** of concussion and complications headache, stupor, apathy, pupillary changes, plantar extensor. LP with fluid pressure but increased protein. Treated by biparietal burr holes and blood is removed by suction.

SAQ 18 What are different types of cerebral herniation?

The major varieties of cerebral herniation are: (i) transtentorial, (ii) foramen magnum, (iii) subfalcine

SAQ 19 What is coning?

Downward herniation of brain through foramen magnum due to raised intracranial pressure.

SAQ 20 What are the signs of a coning?

- Coma
- Hypertension
- Bradycardia
- Unreactive midsize pupil
- Cheyne-Stokes respiration
- Diabetes insipidus due to traction damage of pituitary stalk.

LAQ 21 What are clinical features of anterior, middle and posterior cranial fossa fracture?

Anterior fossa	Middle fossa	Posterior fossa
Escape of cranial content through nose. Nerves affected are 1st, 3rd, 4th, 5th, 6th.	Escapes of cranial content through ear or mouth Nerves affected 7th and 8th.	Extravasation of blood through mastoid or sub-occipital regions, Affects 9–10 and 11th cranial nerves.

LAQ 22 Classify brain tumours.

According to WHO, brain tumours are of following types:

1. Neuroepithelial tumours
   - Glioma
     - Astrocytoma
     - Oligodendroglioma
     - Choroid plexus tumour
     - Ependymoma
   - Pineal tumour
   - Neuronal tumour
     - Ganglioglioma
     - Neuroblastoma
     - Gangliocytoma
2. Nerve sheath tumour (acoustic neuroma)
3. Meningeal tumour (Meningioma)
4. Pituitary tumours
5. Germ cell tumours
   - Germinoma
   - Teratoma
6. Lymphoma
7. Metastatic tumours
8. Contiguous extension of regional tumour

Tumour like malformation

Craniopharyngioma, epidermoid tumour, collection cyst, dermoid tumours

SAQ 23 How is the CSF formed and drained?

About 140 ml of CSF supports, removes end product of metabolism and maintains haemostasis of brain and spinal cord. Rate of production 0.2–0.4 ml/minute, replaced 3 times per day.

Most of the CSF is produced in lateral ventricle, goes to third ventricle via foramen of Monro. From 3rd ventricle via aqueduct to 4th ventricle and via formen of Luscheka (laterally) and Magendie to surface and ultimately reabsorbed via arachnoid villi.

SAQ 24 Define hydrocephalus.

It is disproportionate increased amount of CSF in brain.

LAQ 25 What are the different methods of diagnosing cerebral tumours?

(i) History
(ii) X-ray chest (bronchial carcinoma)
(iii) X-ray skull (silver beaten appearance, separation of sutures, erosion of posterior clinoid process, lateral displacement of calcified pineal shadows, alternate in skull vascular marking, meningioma)
(iv) EEG
(v) LP
(vi) CT scanning
(vii) Arteriography
(viii) Myodil ventriculogram
(ix) Air encephalography
(x) Cerebral puncuture

LAQ 26 What are the causes of SAH?

(i) Rupture aneurysm
(ii) Idiopathic
(iii) AV malformation
(iv) Tumours
(v) Coagulopathy

SAQ 27 What are the different types of surgery done for epilepsy?

(i) If lesions are in amygdala or hippocampus then resection of temporal lobe partially
(ii) Hemidecortication
(iii) Resection of corpus callosum

SAQ 28 Name the conditions which can mimic brain death.

(i) Drug intoxication
(ii) Hypothermia
(iii) Electric shocks injury
(iv) Brainstem encephalitis

SAQ 29 What are the different shunting procedures for hydrocephalus?

These are:

(i) Intracranial shunts connecting ventricle to another intracranial area such as basal cystern
(ii) Ventricular or lumbar shunts diverts CSF to body cavities or right side of heart.

LAQ 30 What are the different tumours of pituitary?

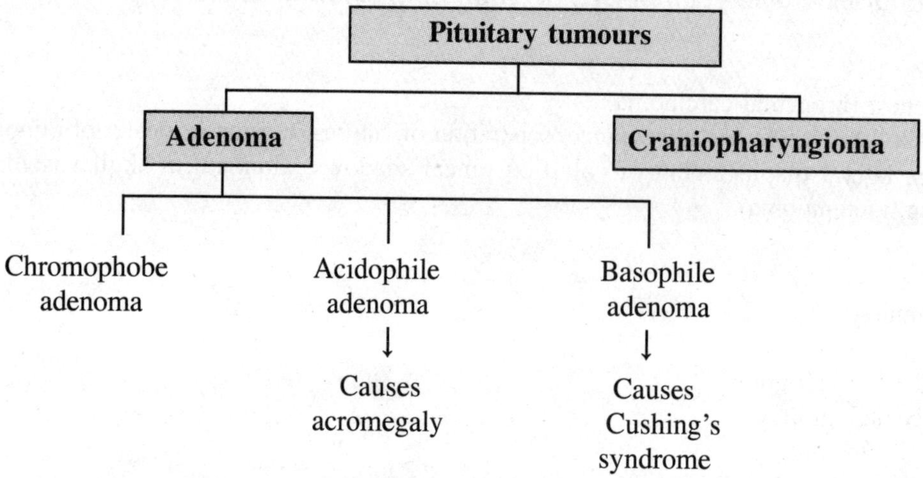

SAQ 31 Mention the indications of surgery in pituitary tumours.

(i) Pressure effect on surrounding
(ii) Inappropriate hormone production not tackleable by drugs.

50 Postoperative Care

SAQ 1 Why the patient needs postoperative care?

The patient needs postoperative case because of:

(i) Breathing problems
(ii) Air passage blockage
(iii) Poor oxygen transport
(iv) Fluid intake and unable to take drugs by mouth
(v) Temperature regulation
(vi) Susceptible to infection

SAQ 2 What are the aims of postoperative care?

(i) Immediate support after surgery
(ii) To relief pain
(iii) To minimize complications
(iv) To review treatment plan (prophylaxis, monitoring contingency)
(v) To maintain team communication

SAQ 3 What are the things to be noted in postoperative patient?

(i) Consciousness
(ii) Cyanosis
(iii) Pain
(iv) Shock
(v) BP
(vi) Dyspnoea
(vii) Temperature
(viii) Hydration
(ix) Pressure area (heels and buttocks)
(x) Infection and discharge

SAQ 4 What is the principle of postoperative fluid therapy?

(i) Maintenance (ii) Replace ongoing loss and (iii) Deficit

SAQ 5 Why postoperative pain management is important?

(i) Humanitarian
(ii) May cause stress
(iii) Pulmonary
(iv) Cardiovascular
(v) Gastrointestinal complications

SAQ 6 What are the different causes of pain in postoperative patient?

(i) Pain at surgical site
(ii) Movement of the wound
(iii) Psychological

SAQ 7 How to write discharge letter?

(i) Name, age and sex of the patient
(ii) Diagnosis
(iii) Treatment
(iv) What to do for complications
(v) Follow up and when to remove stiches

SAQ 8 Name the different drugs used for postoperative pain.

- Paracetamol
- Codeine
- IV or IM morphine
- Aspirin
- NSAID
- Regional block

SAQ 9 When to give frusemide in postoperastive urinary suppression?

It is only given if there is associated CCF.